QUANTUM HEALING

Discover the Power of Self-Healing through the laws of Quantum Physics and the Body-Mind Connection

ADRIAN SATYAM

© Copyright 2019 by Adrian Satyam

All rights reserved.

or blame be held against the publisher for any reparation, damages, or monetary loss due to the information herein, either directly or indirectly.

Respective authors own all copyrights not held by the publisher.

The information herein is offered for informational purposes solely, and is universal as so. The presentation of the information is without contract or any type of guarantee assurance.
The trademarks that are used are without any consent, and the publication of the trademark is without permission or backing by the trademark owner. All trademarks and brands within this book are for clarifying purposes only and are the owned by the owners themselves, not affiliated with this document

Contents

INTRODUCTION...6

CHAPTER 1...9

WHAT IS QUANTUM?...9

CHAPTER 2...33

QUANTUM PHYSICS AND ITS GIFTS TO MEDICINE................33

QUANTUM MIND, MEANING, AND MEDICINE MIND AS SLAYER.............37

THE QUANTUM MECHANICAL HUMAN BODY....................38

THE TRUTH ABOUT OUR DNA.......................................42

ALTERING DNA AND ITS EFFECTS.................................47

CONSEQUENCES OF DNA MISINFORMATION...............53

BALANCING AND HEAL BODY'S STRUCTURE................54

THE EXPERIENCE OF CONSCIOUS INTENTION.............57

CHAPTER 3...65

CELLULAR LEVEL...65

CHAPTER 4...72

MESSENGERS FROM SPACE...72

CHAPTER 5...92

THE QUANTUM MECHANICAL HUMAN BODY....................92

CHAPTER 6...98

THE QUANTUM BODY IS MORE THAN THE PHYSICAL..............98

THE HEALING PATH TO SUPRAMENTAL INTELLIGENCE...........103

WORKING MULTI-DIMENSIONALLY APPLIED KINESIOLOGY (AK) OR MUSCLE TESTING TECHNIQUES....................120

CONCLUSION...139

INTRODUCTION

The term physics immediately fits every time the word quantum comes up. This habit of mind made Quantum Healing a novel and controversial title in 1989, but a valid problem was suggested by its creator, a curious-minded endocrinologist outside Boston. If every atom and molecule in the universe emerges from the quantum field, does this not also mean our bodies are doing so? There's no way the conclusion is true. In that case we have a mechanical quantum body. Dr. Deepak Chopra then concluded that the complexities of the human body, and the mystery of healing in particular, are ultimately submerged in the quantum field.

Nearly thirty years ago very few scientists thought so. Medical schools generally treated the human body as a system that was subdivided into the working parts of a machine — organs, tissues, and cells. The solid was at fault when the body broke down from sickness. Bacteria reached to disrupt an organ's internal function, or a worn-out component failed. An arthritic joint was deemed similar to a tire wearing thin tread.

Modern scientific medicine goes into complex explanation, but ultimately it follows the two fundamental principles that unite all sciences: materialism and reductionism. Materialism holds that every event must have a physical explanation. Reductionism holds that complex issues can be broken down into smaller component parts, with all solutions and answers lying within. Quantum Healing blew the whistle on both principles, not because they are inherently wrong, but because, especially when it came to the human body, they left out certain extremely important things.

Materialism has left out the relation between the mind and the body. Brain is not human. And our emotions allow our bodies to move, something that we take as a matter of course the minute we get out of bed in the morning but it's a great mystery. You can't find the slightest trace of an idea when you split the body down into muscles, tissues, and cells, and yet the mind has to be connected to the body! How?

Reductionism stripped the body of its holistic existence. Trillions of cells are working to support each other, helping to maintain overall health and equilibrium. A microscopic electrical storm produces up to a quadrillion neural connections within the brain, and yet the outcome is thought ordered, not a jumble of static. As qualified as medical science is in dissecting body and brain, it has little to tell about the whole life experience, yet that experience specifically impinges upon who gets sick and who remains healthy.

Deepak wasn't the first to see these flaws and omissions, but Quantum Healing was brave enough to become the first book to propose a road to new answers. He suggested that quantum physics define an unseen world out of which both mind and body arise and join. Quantum Healing struck a nerve by focusing on the medicine's most baffling phenomenon, spontaneous cancer remission. How could a patient's body suddenly disappear from the most intractable illness, the focus of billion-dollar efforts to find a cure? Since oncology is a game of numbers, it was easier to simply ignore such unusual events as exceptions. But if science prides itself on moving wherever nature takes us, the medical journals do well record these situations. We push us to reconsider the whole materialistic, reductionist model — Deepak was happy to go there.

Quantum Therapy was not meant to cure cancer, Alzheimer's or any other intractable illness. This started out to see the human body through smarter eyes, and human existence in general. I am curious about genes and the brain as a scientist; I am totally fascinated by the nature of consciousness as an individual. Quantum Healing galvanized my belief that there's no need to divide these regions. We obviously fit together, and once we feel confident that self-awareness is essential to the body's safe functioning, it will be central to life itself. Beyond that, there are infinite possibilities.

CHAPTER 1

WHAT IS QUANTUM?

Quantum literally means "how great" or "how much," but in fact it represents the smallest discrete unit of the consciousness fluid area. The perception of the subatomic waves of light, sound, and energy gives us the most amazing experience of wholeness, of being completely connected to at-one –atoned with the whole sacred web of life.

Light waves called photons are quanta, brilliant light strands, the string theory "strings." Sound, energy and all life travel in waves as well. The electron spin and wave structure of the quantum waves makes a change as we set a goal. We are sending out reverberations all over the field. There is an intrinsic strength in our life when we are mindful of this realm of wholeness and are grateful for it; there is a profound spiritual liberation open to all.

Existing as both matter and energy in a wave state, as some saints, yogis and others have said, the quanta streaming at its optimum frequency will glow. The whole quantum field is malleable to every one of us feelings, appearance, and purpose.

In Quantum Healing, we merge the personal conscious mind with the super-conscious Mind and train the subconscious mind to share in your Original Gift to the world for the highest good. When we reach wider knowledge fields through Meditation, Yoga, Shamanic Journeying, PSYCH-K, and Creative Practice, we keep a non-dual perspective of reality, experiencing life as a network of intertwined pathways of light, a Loom of Love.

While mainstream psychiatry addresses individual problems and can help solve problems at one point, Energy Therapy and Transpersonal Therapies such as Quantum Healing tackle the many relationships and at-one-offs that promote awareness of who we really are, loving relationships and artistic and spiritual awakenings that bring us to a greater level of consciousness.

THE HIDDEN PHYSIOLOGY

Studies on natural cancer cures, performed in both the USA and Japan, has shown that almost every patient encounters a dramatic shift in consciousness just before the cure occurs. He believes he will be cured, and he thinks the driving power is within himself, but not confined to him— it reaches beyond his personal boundaries, all over nature. Immediately he says, "I'm not just confined to my body. All that happens around me is part of myself. "At that time, it seems that these people are leaping to a higher level of consciousness that prevents the cancer. The cancer cells then either vanish, in some cases literally immediately, or at the very least recover without further affecting the body.

The jump in knowledge seems to be the answer. And it doesn't have to come in a flash. When a physicist talks about such sudden changes the word that comes to mind is quantum. The term signifies a distinct jump from one point to a higher level of functioning— the quantum leap.

Quantum is also a technical term once only accessible to scientists but now rising in common use. Formal, a quantum is "the indivisible unit in which waves can be transmitted or absorbed," as the eminent British scientist Stephen Hawking describes it. The quantum is, in layman's terms, a building block. Light is built up by photons, electricity from the charge of one electron, momentum from the graviton (a potential particle that is not yet found in nature), and so on for all forms of energy— each of them is based on a quantity and cannot be broken down into anything smaller.

Both definitions — a discrete leap to a higher level, and a force's irreducible level. So I want to use the word quantum healing. Although the word is fresh, that is not the concept itself. There were always people who did not follow the normal healing path. Of starters, a tiny minority don't die away from cancer; others have tumors that grow much quicker than their disease numbers suggest. Other remedies with unknown origins— religious regeneration, spontaneous remissions, and the successful use of placebos, or "dummy drugs "— also lead to a quantum leap. Why? For what? Because the staff of inner consciousness seems to have facilitated a dramatic jump— a quantum leap— in the healing process in all these cases.

Consciousness is a power which undervalues most of us. Typically, even in the most painful moments of crisis, we do not center our inner consciousness or use its real power. That may clarify why "miracle" remedies are greeted with a combination of wonder, skepticism and respect. Yet all have consciousness. Such miracles are perhaps variations to natural ability. If your body mends a fractured bone, why isn't that a miracle? It is definitely complicated, far too difficult for medicine to replicate as a healing process; it requires an incredible number of perfectly synchronized processes, of which medicine recognizes only the major ones and those that are incomplete.

The explanation why treating cancer by yourself is a miracle, yet mending a broken arm is not due to the link between the mind and the body: the broken bone seems to mend itself naturally, without the mind's intervention; however, a natural cancer cure, as it is widely believed, relies on a special quality of mind, a profound desire to live, a heroically positive outlook, or some other rare ability. It means there are two forms of recovery, one being natural, the other being uncommon, or at least extraordinary.

That distinction, I think, is false. The broken arm mends when knowledge helps it mend, and the same holds true for the miracle recovery of cancer, the long-term persistence of HIV, the redemption of religion, and even the ability to live to a great old age without falling prey to illness. The explanation why not everyone succeeds in getting the healing process as far as it can go is that we greatly vary in our ability to mobilize it.

We can see this in the way different people are reacting to illness. A minute fraction of all patients who develop an incurable disease fail to recover themselves, far less than 1 per cent. A larger fraction, but still below 5 percent, live much longer than the average— this is reported in 2 percent of AIDS patients who have survived longer than eight years, whereas the vast majority do not survive over two. Such effects are not limited to incurable illnesses. Research has typically shown that with excellent results only 20 per cent of patients with severe yet treatable conditions improve. This leaves about 80 percent who are either not recovered or only partly recovering. Why is ineffective cure so out of proportion so far? Who sets a survivor apart from a non-survivor?

The good patients have apparently learned to inspire their own recovery, and the most successful ones have gone much further than that. They consider quantum healing key. We are the genies of the link between mind and body. Modern medicine cannot even attempt to replicate its treatments, because no treatment that depends on medication or anesthesia is paced so perfectly, so wonderfully organized, so safe and free of side effects, so effortless as theirs. Their ability springs from such a deep level that you can go no deeper. If we knew what their minds were doing to fuel their bodies, then we would have in our hands the basic unit of the healing process.

As yet, medicine has not taken the quantum leap, and the word *quantum* has no clinical application. Because quantum physics works with ultra-high-speed accelerators, you may think that quantum healing uses radioisotopes or X rays. But that is the opposite of what it means.

Quantum healing pushes toward the very heart of the mind-body system away from traditional, high-tech processes. It's that heart where healing starts. To go there and learn to facilitate the healing process, you need to get through all of the body's grosser levels—cells, bodies, organs, to systems — and hit the intersection point of mind and matter, the place where consciousness actually begins to have an impact.

More can be said in terms of consciousness influencing the body, to the point that over the past few decades the distance between "natural" healing and "miraculous" healing has been narrowing even more. As for mainstream medicine, the main obstacle is a firm belief that the body works fully like a physical machine. If that were so, then the experiment below would have failed.

The experiment was the brainchild of Harvard psychologist Ellen Langer's pioneering work, which explored the idea of aging having a major mental component as far back as 1981. (The idea is in fact ancient in nature. Classical Indian mystic and guru Adi Shankara declared that people were growing older and dying because they saw other people grow older and die.) In 1981, Langer took eight men in their seventies, all in good health but displaying signs of age, and submerged them in an experience that was like time travel back to 1959, with music. The people were told to act as if they were their younger self, as Langer had already done tests in which memory loss in the elderly could sometimes be overcome by providing an opportunity to recall the subjects. Or put it another way, the mind was driven or influence the body.

The men were checked on different aging measures such as grip strength, flexibility and how well they could hear and see before reaching the time-capsule area. The party had gained on seven out of eight tests at the end of the five days, including better vision, a surprising revelation. Both looked younger than outside jurors had determined. Thirty-three years ago Langer continued more or less intuitively, without the awareness of gene expression and neuroplasticity that we can turn to today (more about those breakthroughs in later parts of "Expanding the Topic").

Langer moved into a retirement home in another surprising trial, splitting her subjects into two classes. Some houseplants had been offered to both for their space. One party was advised they were responsible for keeping the plants alive, and in their own daily schedule, they could make choices. The other party was told the workers should tend the gardens, and they were given no choice about their set daily schedule, however. Twice as many participants in the first group were still alive at the end of eighteen months compared to the second group. (The same logic is behind the agreed practice of giving the aged a pet to look after. At the very least it increases their morale and quality of life. It can also extend their lives.)

Aging and healing have in common that they have long been seen as fixed mechanisms based on rigid physical limitations. The equation never included an unseen aspect like making your own decisions about how to spend your day. This tendency has been changing for quite some time, but when Quantum Healing emerged, only the early signs became evident. What's important today isn't the recognition of consciousness as a healing factor— that war has been fought, more or less. Alternatively, we need a set of new ideas as to how far understanding can go in improving healing and aging, not to mention intractable chronic pain, addictions, dependency on prescription drugs, recovery from surgery, etc.

Benefits of Quantum Healing

- Works on all levels – physical, emotional, psychological, spiritual and soul level
- Helps to heal from an illness
- Releases old traumas, guilt, vows, curses
- Heals family karma and past lives
- Heals relationships
- Helps to get rid of obsessions and negative patterns
- Works on the level of DNA; healing genetic issues
- Helps abundance and deserving
- Helps spiritual growth and directs toward the soul's purpose

THE BODY CANNOT BE CONTROLLED

For regular practice the doctor goes back to his work once the operation is over, with his normal ideas. But even those, the medical school's stock-in-trade, have buckled. To give just one example: medicine has accepted the degeneration of brain function in the elderly as a natural occurrence since its inception as a field of rational scientific study. This deterioration was thoroughly documented with "hard" findings— as we age, our brains are shrinking, growing lighter, and annually losing millions of neurons. We have our full neuronal complement by age 2, and the number starts to decrease by age 30. Every single brain cell death is permanent, as neurons do not recover. Based on this well-known fact, brain aging appears to be scientifically valid; unfortunately but eventually, growing old would result in loss of memory, diminished ability to reason, reduced comprehension, and associated symptoms.

Nevertheless, these time-honored beliefs have now proved to be wrong. Careful study of stable elderly people— as compared to the ill, disabled people who usually studied medicine — revealed that 80% of older Americans, barring psychological distress (such as isolation, sadness, or lack of external stimulation), do not experience significant memory deficits as they mature. The ability to retain new information may decrease, which is why older people are forgetting phone numbers, addresses, and the need to go into a room; but the ability to remember past events, called long-term memory, is actually improving. (One authority on aging quotes Cicero, who declared, "I have never heard of an old man who forgot where his money was hidden.") In tests where 70-year-olds matched 20-year-olds, older people performed better in this area of memory than the younger ones. By training the other form of memory— called short-term memory— for a few minutes each day, the older group could almost suit the younger participants, who were at their peak mental function.

Maybe we should expand the "prime of life." The key, as with almost any other "normal" regression in old age, relies on mental habits, not on nervous system circuitry. So long as a person stays mentally active, he will remain as intellectual as in middle age and youth. During their lives, humans will still kill over one billion neurons at an average rate of 18 million per year, but this deficit is accounted for by another component, the branch-like filaments called dendrites, which link the nerve cells.

A nerve cell appears to be highly individual in nature, but it usually has a central bulbous segment from which thin arms radiate, like a fruit. Such limbs, or axons, end in a spiral of tiny filaments that seemed treelike to the early anatomists, and they called them dendrites for "rock" after the Greek word. Dendrites, which can range in number from less than a dozen to more than a thousand per cell, function as contact points, allowing the neuron to send signals to its neighbors. Through growing new dendrites, a neuron will open up new communication channels in all directions, like a switchboard that sprouts extra lines.

It is unknown how a thought is actually formed between brain cells or how the bewilderingly vast number of connections interrelate — millions of dendrites come together at major junction points in the body, such as the solar plexus, not to mention the billions to billions in the brain itself. Yet studies have shown that new dendrites will grow up to advanced old age all the way through life. The current view is that we easily get the physical structure for unimpaired brain function from this new growth. Senility is not Physically natural in a healthy brain. A rich multiplication of dendrites could even lie behind growing wise in old age, a time when more and more of life is being seen in its totality— in other words, more interconnected, just as the nerve cells are more interconnected through their new dendrites.

This example shows how fundamentally mistaken science can be if it believes it is superior to intellect. It may be true to say a nerve cell generates ideas, but it is equally true to say that thinking produces nerve cells. In the case of the new dendrites, the new tissue is produced by the habit of thinking, remembering and being mentally active. This is no single observation, either. Curiously enough, as soon as the idea of the "new old age" became acceptable in physicians ' minds, our perceptions of many aspects of degeneration began to change.

For starters, as long as you exercise, the musculature of your body will not wither, and your energy will remain unimpaired of life, even though endurance will gradually diminish. When 65 you should qualify for a marathon, as long as you are in good physical shape and exercise sensitively. Likewise, the heart grows with age, becoming less resilient and circulating fewer blood each minute, but heart disease and artery hardening, thought to be absolutely normal with old age a few decades ago, are now believed to be avoidable, based on diet and lifestyle too. Due to better management of hypertension and less obesity in our diets, strokes, another granted in old age, have decreased by 40 per cent just in the last decade. A significant percentage of "inevitable" senility was linked to vitamin deficiency, poor diet, and dehydration. The overall result of these results is a dramatic reconsideration of old age; a less obvious result is that the whole body has to be rethought at any stage of life.

What's happening in medicine on every front is that the healthy body is proving to be more robust and flexible than expected up to now. Although medical school teaches that germ A triggers disease B and is treated with drug C, nature seems to believe that among others, this is just one choice. A decade ago, for example, the behavioral solution to cancer treatment would have been mocked. Yet, by using feelings, patients do seem to be able to participate in their cancer treatment, and even control the progression of the illness. A 61-year-old man with throat cancer approached Dr. O. Carl Simonton, a radiologist at the University of Texas, in 1971. The illness advanced very far; the patient could hardly chew, and his weight had fallen to 98 pounds.

Not only was the prognosis extremely poor— the doctors gave him a 5 per cent chance to survive five years following treatment— but the patient was already so frail that it seemed impossible he would respond well to chemotherapy, which is the normal medicine for this disease. Dr. Simonton proposed in frustration, but also intrigued to seek a psychological approach, that the man improve his radiation therapy by using imagination. He's been taught how to treat his cancer as clearly as possible. He was then asked to imagine his immune system using any mental picture that applied to him, as the white blood cells successfully attacked the cancer cells and washed them out of the body, leaving only healthy cells behind.

The guy said he saw his immune cells as a white-particle blizzard, covering the tumor like snow surrounding a black rock. Dr Simonton made him go home and replicate this vision throughout the day at intervals. The guy agreed, and his tumor quickly seemed to dwindle. It was definitely smaller in a couple of weeks, and his reaction to radiation was nearly free of side effects; the tumor was gone after two months.

Needless to say, Dr. Simonton was confused and puzzled, even though the psychological approach had been so strong. How to beat a cancer cell by a thought? The mechanism was completely unknown — in reality, the process might be unknowable considering the fiendish nature of the immune system and the nervous system, both of which were obviously involved here. The recipient, for his part, welcomed his cure without undue shock. He told Dr. Simonton that arthritis in his legs stopped him from doing as much stream-fishing as he wished. Now that the cancer has gone away, why not continue to imagine the arthritis too? This is exactly what happened in a couple more weeks ' time. For a follow-up span of six years the man remained free from both cancer and arthritis.

This now-famous case is a milestone in mind-body therapy but it's not the whole story, sadly. Visualization treatment by Dr. Simonton (it has branched out into a large mind-body program) does not consistently cure cancer. One of my patients actually used it to heal herself from breast cancer, I agree, even though she was using the procedure on her own and not under the supervision of a doctor. Nevertheless, long-term statistical studies question whether such intermittent outcomes are better than conventional treatment ones.

There is a major difference nowadays in traditional therapy. Of example, if a woman with breast cancer discovers the tumor while it is still very low and isolated, the odds of healing her (a "cure" means living without a recurrence of the disease for at least three years) actually exceed 90 percent. In contrast, the number of spontaneous remissions would be well below 1/10 of 1 per cent, at the most generous estimate. It will not become the medication of choice until a psychiatric or other alternative therapy outperforms radiation and chemotherapy. Although patients may be hoping for such strategies, the majority of doctors often fear and distrust them.

But even though Dr. Simonton's patient was one of a sort, he's enough to shake our comprehension of how the body heals itself, because here's nature finding a way to battle mortality that no doctor has tried — and here's also the grim chance that what the doctor usually does isn't saving nature, yet stifling it.

Over the last decade, fascinated and innovative clinicians have flocked to experiment with mind-body technologies, from biofeedback and hypnotism to visualizations and behavioral change. The findings were amorphous across the board, and difficult to interpret. Psychologist Michael Lerner spent three years conducting a thorough study of forty hospitals offering alternative treatments to cancer, the techniques of which varied from plants and macrobiotics to visualizing positive mental images. He found that these "complementary cancer centers" were sought by patients who were generally well-educated and prosperous, that the doctors running the clinics were also serious and well-intentioned, but that wherever he visited, nothing near a cancer cure had been discovered.

A fairly large proportion (40 percent) when interviewing the patients felt they had experienced at least a slight improvement in the quality of their lives. Another 40% reported actual medical improvements in their condition, lasting from a couple of days to a number of years. At the opposite ends of the spectrum, only 10 percent fell, one group claiming they received nothing from the procedure and the other that they were now partially or completely healed from their disease. The experience of alternative approaches suggests typically that they provide patients with a degree of relaxation and recovery, but disappointingly, the levels of remission are not radically different from those of conventional therapy.

There are other issues that run deeper than inconsistent results: the study of the mind-body appears to be afflicted by an inability to justify its basic principle rigorously, that the mind affects the body to either health or illness. It seems completely self-evident that sick people and healthy people enjoy different mental states, but the causal connection remains elusive. A new breast cancer study conducted at the University of Pennsylvania in 1985 failed to find any correlation between patients ' mental attitude and their ability to escape their illness after two years. The whole idea of feelings influencing cancer was rejected in an editorial following the report which appeared in the influential New England Journal of Medicine. "Our confidence in illness as a direct reflection of mental states," declared the editorial, "is essentially myth." In addition, letters deluged the magazine, most of them from physicians who strongly disagreed with the interpretation of the editorial. Discounting mental behavior as a factor of sickness definitely sounds irrational, much less so than myths. Every practitioner knows that the will of the patient to recover plays a vital part in his treatment. Wedded to "strong" treatment, most physicians can nevertheless accept the idea that mentality, conviction and feelings do not play their part. At the dawn of Western medicine, Hippocrates claimed that "a patient who is mortally ill may yet recover from his doctor's confidence in the goodness." This has been corroborated by several modern studies, showing that people who trust their doctor and yield to his care are more likely to recover than those who treat treatment with distrust, anxiety and antagonism.

Tempers erupted in the aftermath of the editorial and lines of loyalty were drawn, while the issues became even more confused. Three independent mid-1980s surveys on breast cancer survival rates came up with three completely different findings. In one, the people that showed strong positive attitudes seemed to outlive those who were pessimistic, and it didn't matter because their cancers were more advanced — positive emotions, it seemed, helped them survive from a late-stage metastasized cancer, whereas those with negative emotions died from tiny tumors that had been detected relatively early.

Nevertheless, a second study showed that any positive disposition, if conveyed rather than held back, led to the survival of this very deadly illness. While the first observation confirms common sense— the concept that positivity is better than depression— the second does much the same from another perspective, the principle being that battle is better than giving up. A so-called cancer identity, which sucks up feelings and somehow turns anger into malignant cells, was given attention. The opposite would be the type of "strong will to live," which can either be positive or negative.

All of this followed a certain rationale, except for the research that seemed to begin with in the New England Journal of Medicine, seconded by accompanying studies that found no correlation over two years between any emotional trend and surviving breast cancer. The idea of mind-body medicine was shook, even as it grew in popularity and became one of the most successful advances since the Salk vaccine. Today, a familiar pattern has emerged, in which the public is told of some elating achievement, accompanied by troubling clinical outcomes generally known only in limited medical circles.

A classic example of this was the division of heart attack patients into high-risk Type A personalities and low-risk Type B's, more than three-quarters of them middle-aged males. The Type A personality was meant to be a hard-driving, compulsive man, continually chasing schedules and churning his body of stress hormones, as opposed to the calm, accommodating, more controlled Type B. Type A endured "the illness of being in a hurry;" therefore it was inevitable that his heart would ultimately rebel, leading to a coronary.

Unfortunately, controlled studies have shown that widely accepted distinction is not as smooth as that. It points out that most individuals have some Type A in them and some Type B, and that pain management varies widely, with some classes saying that they excel thereon. Ultimately, a study in 1988 showed that if a man does have a heart attack, Type A recovers more than Type B's. Once the coronary arrives, their desire to excel evidently becomes a gain.

The intricacies of the relationship between mind and body were not to be overcome with ease. If one questions why a healthy attitude cannot be readily associated with good health— it seems to be one of life's most obvious facts— the response has to do first of all with what you mean by "mentalism." This problem is not a metaphysical one but a realistic one. If a patient has cancer, is his mental state determined by how he feels on diagnosis day, months before, or long after? Dr. Lawrence LeShan, founder of the seminal research that associated feelings with cancer in the 1950s, went back to the origins of cancer patients to find the black seed that infected their psyche and he theorized that it lay dormant in the subconscious for years until their illness was triggered.

Resonance

The seemingly simple feature of resonance is indeed a mystery and a wonder. All people and particles dance to its power, from the galaxies to the subatomic.

If both a piano and a guitar were in tune and a G was played on the piano, that would also vibrate the G string on the guitar. Sound waves which move the air transfer the acoustic energy from the piano to the guitar. Similarly, tuned oscillators, that is to say things that can vibrate at the same frequency, require very little effort to transfer energy from one to the other. In this case, the string on the guitar absorbs the piano's energy waves, as it is tuned to the same frequency. Each time oscillators are similarly tuned they form what's called a resonant structure. The string of a guitar and a piano resonates with each other.

If grandfather-type pendulum clocks were mounted against a wall with their pendulums swinging out of phase to each other, their pendulums would lock into phase and beat together in a matter of days. In this scenario, it would be enough energy transmitted through the common wall to cause the clocks to come into sync with each other. This is entrainment, a process that allows two closely tuned devices to coordinate their movement and energy in a rhythm and step match. This phenomenon occurs in the telecommunications industry as well. If you have similarly tuned oscillating circuits which vibrate at similar frequencies, the slower circuit will rise to suit the faster one's speed. We can see in both of these examples how energy is transferred from one similarly tuned system into another.

What is it we should expect from all this? First, when two systems oscillate at different frequencies, an impelling force called resonance exists which causes the two to transfer energy from one to the other. There is another aspect of this energy transfer called entrainment when two similarly tuned systems vibrate at different frequencies which causes them to line up and vibrate at the same frequency. Entraining is the mechanism whereby objects sync their action and energy to fit in rhythm and step together. That also appears to work with biological systems. In many parts of the world, on warm nights, fireflies gathered in a tree will light up by accident. They'll both switch on and off their lights in a coordinated manner before long. I've heard crickets or frogs often all find the same rhythm and coordinate their sounds to each other. In these cases, nature finds it useful or perhaps economical to train the individuals rhythmically.

Perhaps through a more mystical mechanism, women who have shared a house or dormitory over time will discover that their menstrual cycles will also join rhythmically. Scientists have found that even disincarnated animal hearts will enter when kept alive in a laboratory and placed close to each other - the individual hearts will begin to beat in unison. The method is almost identical.

When two things vibrate through resonance and entraining at different frequencies, either the lower vibration will come up, the higher vibration will come down, or they will meet in the middle. Through Quantum-healing, practitioners learn to lift the pulse in their hands to a very high frequency through relaxation and breathing techniques. If they put their hands near someone else who is in distress, the body of their person resonates and reaches into the hands of the patient, like a finely tuned wire. Love is the fundamental pulse allowing individuals to transfer healing energy from one to the other.

The practitioner holds the highest vibration they can when working with Quantum-Healing which becomes the dominant frequency. The "healer" (otherwise known as the client or patient), that is, the person whose body is healing, must actually go in with the practitioner's pulse and suit it. A spiritual teacher named Lazaris has said, "The concept of a great healer is one who was very ill and quickly got better." I believe anyone who claims to be able to cure others is either naive, wrong, narcissistic or insane. All they do is provide the resonant energies that will help others to heal themselves.

The practitioner simply holds a tremendously powerful harmonizing energy, and matches that vibration to the client. The person's inherent body knowledge consuming the energy will do whatever the body finds helpful to promote healing. With an inscrutable level of intelligence the body heals itself. Western civilization sometimes takes for granted the inherent healing ability of the body but it is the ultimate healer. Looking at our body's cells, we see that we have hundreds of billions of cells which constantly feed on oxygen and the food we eat, and release carbon dioxide and other waste materials. Such cells are also concerned with replication and self-healing, with thousands of microscopic changes happening every minute of every day! It's a good thing that I don't have to keep track of all this activity because I have to wonder where I left my keys.

Without the breathing and meditative techniques learned in Quantum-healing, a practitioner can actually descend to the client's vibration and thus get drained from the experience. In Quantum-healing this does not occur as long as we use the techniques to hold a naturally high resonance.

Every single one of us is awash at every moment in the endless stream of life-force energy that passes through and around our bodies. Like the fish that have no understanding of nature, it was only modern Western cultures that rejected life force presence. To acknowledge its existence, everything must be measurable according to the rules inherent in the scientific method. Because scientists don't have enough sensitive instrumentation to quantify or verify life-force presence, they dispute it is possible. This is like rejecting a television channel's presence because that station is not provided by your unit. It's also like rejecting love's presence, because you can't measure its duration or weigh it on a scale.

Life-force is the energy that separates the living from the non-living. It is the animating current of life recognized, appreciated and utilized for thousands of years by numerous cultures around the world. The Chinese call it "Chi" and the Japanese call it "Ki." Both nations and many others use the force for various techniques of soothing massage, acupuncture, and many types of martial arts. The Indian yogis called the energy "Prana" and used their understanding to attain higher levels of consciousness through their yoga, pranayama, meditation, and various practices of healing. It was referred to by the Hawaiian Kahunas as "Mana," and also used for hands-on healing, distant healing, and prayer.

The irony is that in reality every minute of each day all people feel the life-force inside them. We just don't know we are thinking it. For most of us, life-force energy sensations may be analogous to the background noise from the street we live in. We've become so thoroughly used to it that we don't consider it any more. We just hear the noise from the street as we stop and pay close attention to it. Often, the very last things to be seen or noticed are the most blatant and clear. Life-force is just that. But despite the lack of life-force knowledge, it's quickly sensed without much effort by most people. We just need to be able to seek it out.

There may be some sort of intuitive understanding of life-force and Prana, even within English. When someone dies and their vitality and life-force leaves the body, we say the person has "expired." Similarly, when someone experiences a marvelous creative flow, we describe them as being "inspired." To "inspire" and "expire" are the same words we use to describe breathing, and breathing happens to be Prana's primary source. To sum up, life-force energy is the animating current of life functioning with an intelligence level which boggles human imagination. All living things are permeated by Life-force.

Quantum-Healing Principles

- Love is a universal vibration; love communicates with all species, functions at every level and expresses our true nature. It is the foundation of all of life-force healing and the core essence.
- It is common for all people to be able to assist with healing.
- Healing is a teachable skill that grows stronger with practice. In the course of time, practitioners become stronger in running the energy and in their healing capacity.
- Thinking carries on from power. To create a high-energy field, the practitioner uses aim and various meditations and uses the environment to cover the area to be healed.
- Resonance and entrainment cause the healed area to change its vibration to match the practitioner's. The patient simply takes the new echo up and holds it.
- Absolutely no one else can recover. The healer is the person in need of cure. The practitioner just holds a resonance to let the body heal itself.

- It's important to trust the cycle. The work can cause temporary pain or other distressing symptoms all of which are part of healing. The life force and the cycle of regeneration work with depth and insight that are beyond our creation and comprehension.
- The strength suits the body's natural wisdom to do the requisite remedy. The practitioner pays attention to "intelligence about the body" and "chases the pain."
- By doing the practice the patient often provides relief.
- Breathing amplifies the power of life.
- The application of relaxation and yoga exercises helps the energy focus, which many times enhances the power, like a laser.
- Synergy is the result of working together with several healers and increases the sum of the pieces. It could be very effective.
- Each person's gifts are unique in life and healing. Some people are particularly gifted in treating particular conditions.
- Healing can be performed from a distance and can be very effective.
- Quantum-Touch blends many curing modalities easily and effectively.
- The desire to communicate with one's faith, in whatever shape it is considered to be, and to ask for help brings to this research another layer of influence.

CHAPTER 2

QUANTUM PHYSICS AND ITS GIFTS TO MEDICINE

1. Improved disease screening and treatment

Using a relatively new technique known as the bio-barcode test, scientists can now use gold nanoparticles to detect disease-specific signs, or "biomarkers," in our blood, which are visible using MRI imaging and have special quantum properties that allow them to bind to disease-fighting cells. Such nanoparticles of gold are completely safe for human consumption. This approach is also less costly, more versatile and more accurate than traditional alternatives.

Mikhail Lukin, a Harvard physics professor and pioneer in quantum optics and atomic physics, also focuses on engineering nanoscale diamond particles for similar purposes. He aims to potentially use non-toxic diamond particles to take images of human cells from within and to diagnose illness without exposing patients to radiation.

By allowing ultra-precise measurements, Quantum sensors can also improve the MRI machine itself. Instead of the whole body, a new form of quantum-based MRI could be used to look at single molecules or groups of molecules, offering physicians a far more accurate image.

Many quantum based approaches for treating diseases are also being developed. For example, gold nanoparticles can be "programmed" to build up in tumor cells only, allowing accurate imaging as well as tumor laser destruction without destroying healthy cells.

2. **No more needles**

University of York researchers have developed a pad that can be added to the skin to administer tailored treatments without hypodermic needles. The pad, dubbed the Nanject, will be used without damaging healthy cells to distribute cancer drugs.

Here's how it works: before being inserted into the bloodstream, the nanoparticles are covered in antigens (substances that bind to antibodies) where they bind to cancer cells. The patient is then placed in an MRI machine which causes the particles to heat up and destroy the cancer cells. The ions cool back down when the unit is switched off, and can be withdrawn from the body without hurting the user.

Needle-phobic patients can also be excited about this kind of progression: the Nanject patch substitutes a single syringe with many tiny ones consisting of polymer nanofilaments that distribute the drug by hair follicles.

However, the nanotech drug delivery route has another, perhaps more important benefit: it removes some of the toughest barriers to medication distribution, especially in remote and impoverished areas. There is no need for a qualified nurse or surgeon to deliver drugs with a patch; it is self-administered by anyone through a procedure that is as easy as putting on a band-aid. Nanotech drug delivery also allows lower doses, as nanoparticles are not consumed like pill-based medicines by stomach acid. Finally, medications such as the Nanject can help prevent disease transmission by unsterilized needles–a major problem in developing nations.

3. Hacking human biology

Quantum mechanics has the ability to provide us with more knowledge about human biology beyond better disease detection and highly targeted, needle-free therapies.

Australian scientists have recently discovered a way to investigate a living cell's inner workings using a new method of laser microscopy based on the concepts of quantum mechanics. And we can use quantum computers to sequence DNA quickly then solve other health-care challenges with Big Data. This opens the possibility of specialized treatment, based on the unique genetic structure of people.

4. More secure health data

For obvious reasons people want to protect their health data, so it's important to consider all the ways it can be compromised. For example, in the future, hackers may become able to intercept messages retroactively.

One of the attendees of the quantum meeting, Nicolas Gisin, is collaborating with ID Quantique, a company that uses the peculiar properties of quantum phenomena to secure our data in an ultra-safe way. Using quantum entanglement in one of the most practical applications of the technology to date, quantum cryptography prohibits anybody other than the intended recipient from accessing the results. ID Quantique already provides banks and governments with protection, and ultimately sees strong potential in the healthcare sector.

Innovations based on quantum mechanics principles have the potential to affect health care at almost any level, from diagnosis and treatment to data storage and transmission. We need to keep a close eye on quantum science and healthcare— a field that will benefit from increased support for R&D. We are on the cusp of some fascinating developments, and we should all be educating ourselves on how quantum science in the not-so-distant future can change the health care.

QUANTUM MIND, MEANING, AND MEDICINE MIND AS SLAYER

Quantum mind (sometimes referred to as quantum consciousness) is the belief that consciousness involves quantum processes, as opposed to the concept of conventional neurobiology in which the operation of the brain is entirely classical, and quantum processes play no role in computation.

While many attempts at a theory of quantum consciousness are pseudoscientific by naively believing that the strangeness of quantum mechanics is similar to the strangeness of consciousness, more advanced theories of quantum consciousness are an attempt to solve the "combination question;" the problem that describes how a network of classical neurons can combine to form a single subject of experience Nevertheless, no experimental evidence of computationally important quantum processes is currently available in the human brain, partly due to the technical difficulty of studying the brain at adequate spatial and temporal granularity.

Quanta and consciousness

Not all quantum mechanical interpretations assume that quantum collapse occurs, but one of many competing theories about how it occurs is that consciousness causes collapse, if it does. Since these ideas focused on consciousness were developed, this form of quantum physics has been drawn by people who want to believe that consciousness is in some way special. Several followers to quantum physics focused on supernatural consciousness were woo-meisters and pseudoscientists who often suggested costly solutions to problems. Despite this also attracted respected scientists such as Eugene Wigner to quantum consciousness, a view which Wigner later repudiated. It is difficult for lay people to see at the present level of knowledge how far quantum consciousness is a reasonable theory, and how much it is wishful thinking. However, it should be noted that unless substance dualism is true, which most scientists doubt, it should be possible for conscious minds to collapse wave functions just as much as unconscious photodetectors can. If this were not the case, it would mean that our minds are composed of some non-physical material which does not make up implicit photodetectors.

THE QUANTUM MECHANICAL HUMAN BODY

"I can't define the real problem, and I believe there's no real problem, but I'm not confident there's no real problem." Richard Feynman, an American scientist, said this about the infamous problems and paradoxes in quantum mechanics, scientists use theory to explain the smallest objects in the world. But he might as well have spoken of the equally knotty consciousness issue.

Some scientists believe that we already understand what awareness is, or that it is a mere illusion. But many others feel that we have not grasped where consciousness actually comes from.

The persistent mystery of consciousness has even prompted some scholars to invoke for clarification in quantum physics. The idea has always been met with skepticism which is not surprising: answering one mystery with another does not sound wise. Yet certainly, these concepts are not irrational and neither are they random.

As one aspect the imagination seemed to force its way into early quantum theory, to the great discomfort of physicists. What's more, quantum computers are predicted to be able to accomplish things ordinary computers can't accomplish, which reminds us how our brains can accomplish things that are beyond artificial intelligence yet. "Quantum consciousness" as a mystical woo is widely derided, but it just won't go away.

Quantum mechanics is the best theory we have to describe the world of atoms and subatomic particles at the nuts-and-bolts stage. Perhaps the most renowned of its mysteries is the fact that a quantum experiment's outcome can change depending on whether or not we choose to measure some property of the involved particles.

When the early pioneers of quantum theory first noticed that "observer effect," they were deeply troubled. It seemed to contradict the fundamental assumption behind all science: that there is an empirical universe out there, whoever we may be. If the way the universe conducts depends on how −or if −we look at it, what can we mean by "reality?"

Many scientists now believe that, whether consciousness affects quantum mechanics or not, it may really occur because of it. They think quantum theory may be necessary to fully understand how the brain functions.

Could it be that just as physical phenomena can seem to be in two positions at once, so can a quantum brain hang on to two concepts which are mutually contradictory at the same time?

These ideas are speculative and it may turn out that for or in the workings of the mind, quantum physics has no fundamental role. But if nothing else, then these possibilities show just how strangely we are forced to think by quantum theory.

In the "double-slit experiment" comes the most famous intrusion of the mind into quantum mechanics. Imagine shining a beam of light on a screen featuring two parallel slits which are closely spaced. Some of the light goes through the slits, whereupon another screen strikes.

Light can be seen as a kind of stream, and when waves appear from two such slits they can interact with one another. They reinforce each other if their peaks coincide, whereas if a peak and a trough coincide, they cancel off. Such wave distortion is called diffraction, which creates a pattern of alternating bright and dark lines on the rear panel, where the light waves are either amplified or canceled out.

This phenomenon was known to be a feature of wave behavior more than 200 years ago, well before the existence of quantum theory.

It is also possible to perform the double slit experiment with quantum particles such as electrons; tiny charged particles which are components of atoms. Such particles will act like waves in a counter-intuitive twist. That means when a stream of them passes through the two slits, they can undergo diffraction, producing an interference pattern.

Now assume the quantum particles are sent one by one through the slits, and their appearance at the frame is also seen one by one. Now there seems to be nothing to interact with each particle along its path–yet the sequence of particle impacts that build up over time shows bands of interference.

The implication appears to be that each particle passes through both slits at the same time and interferes with itself. This "both paths at once" combination is known as superposition state.

When we put a detector inside or just behind one crack, we will figure out whether or not some single particle is going through it. However, in that case the interference vanishes. Just by following the direction of a particle–even if that observation should not affect the motion of the particle–we are modifying the result.

The physicist Pascual Jordan, who collaborated with quantum mystic Niels Bohr in the 1920s in Copenhagen, put it this way: "observations not only disrupt what needs to be measured, they create it... we compel[a quantum particle] to assume a definite position." In other words, Jordan said, "we produce the results of measurements ourselves."

THE TRUTH ABOUT OUR DNA

But we are bringing with us signs of those other animals. There are remnants of genetic material from a number of ancient humans hidden within our DNA that no longer exist. Such signs indicate a long history of intermingling as our direct ancestors met ancient humans— and paired them with them. Since we are using increasingly complex technologies to study these genetic connections, we are learning not only about these extinct humans but also about the broader picture of how we have evolved as a species.

Joshua Akey, a professor at the Lewis-Sigler Institute for Integrative Genomics, is at the forefront of efforts to understand this wider picture. He calls his research method genetic archaeology, and the way we learn about our past is transforming. "We will excavate various human forms not from soil and fossils but directly from DNA," he said.

Combining his experience in genetics and Darwinian evolution with quantitative and mathematical techniques, Akey explores the evolutionary links between modern humans and two groups of extinct hominids: Neanderthals, paleoanthropology's original "cave men;" and Denisovans, an early human recently discovered. Akey's research reveals a dynamic history of early human intermingling, which is representative of several centuries of worldwide population changes.

"There is often a difference between the researchers who go out and gather unusual samples and the researchers who do really innovative theory and data analysis, and he did both," said Kelley Harris, a former colleague of Akey's who is now an assistant professor of genome sciences at Washington University.

Like many of us, Akey's long been involved in the evolution of the human race. "People want their history to be remembered," he said. "But even more so we want to know what it means to be alive." Akey continued this fascination during his education. In the late 1990s, during his graduate work at the University of Texas Health Science Center in Houston, he looked at how contemporary human beings in different parts of the world were genetically related to each other, and used early gene sequencing methods to try to understand these relations.

Gene sequencers are devices which specify the order of the four chemical bases that make up the DNA molecule (A, T, C, and G). Analysts can classify the genetic information found in a strand of DNA by determining the sequence of those bases.

Nevertheless, gene sequencing research has been making dramatic headway since the 1990s. A new technology known as sequencing of the next generation came into use around 2010 and allowed researchers to analyze a very significant number of genetic variations in the human genome. It took ten years to sequence the first human genome, but in just a matter of hours, these new machines receive entire genome sequence data from thousands of individuals. "When the next-generation sequencing techniques started to become the dominant force in genetics," Akey said, "it changed the whole field completely. How revolutionary this development has been is hard to overestimate. "The size of the data that can now be processed has allowed researchers to answer a whole slew of new questions that would not have been feasible with the previous technologies.

Another such concern is the relationship between modern humans and ancient humans, including Neanderthals. In addition, this issue fostered a vigorous debate over whether modern humans were bearing Neanderthal genes. Researchers ' opinions-both pro and con-ticked back and forth like a metronome for many years.

Gradually, however, a few researchers— including geneticists Svante Pääbo from the Max Planck Institute in Germany and his colleague Richard (Ed) Green from the University of California-Santa Cruz — began to show strong evidence that gene transfers from Neanderthals to modern humans had indeed existed. Such researchers estimated in a 2010 study that individuals with non-African descent had a Neanderthal heritage of about 2 per cent.

Since dying out around 30,000 years ago, Neanderthals lived in a large geographical area throughout Europe, the Near East and Central Asia. They lived alongside anatomically modern humans, which evolved around 200,000 years ago in Africa. The archeological record shows that Neanderthals were experts at producing stone tools and developed a number of physical characteristics that specifically suited them to harsh, dark environments such as long noses, thick body hair and large eyes.

Coming on the heels of Neanderthal work by Pääbo and Green, Akey and a friend, Benjamin Vernot, published a paper in Science aimed at retrieving Neanderthal genomes from the modern human genome. A parallel paper was published in Nature by Harvard University's geneticist David Reich, and the two papers together provided the first evidence using the current genome to explore our association with Neanderthals.

Using the genetic variation of current societies to learn about things that have happened in the past means scrutinizing the modern human genome for gene sequences that exhibit characteristics thought to be inherited from a particular type of human being. The sequences are then taken by Akey and his collaborators and linked to the Neanderthal genome, searching for a match.

Using this approach, Akey was able to uncover, on a previously unconceived scale, a complex human history of genetic interconnections. When reported, while the evidence available shows that non-Africans have about 2 percent of Neanderthal genes, Africans, previously believed to have no links with Neanderthals, currently have only 0.5 percent of Neanderthal genes. Scientists have also shown that the Neanderthal gene has led to various diseases seen in modern human societies, such as diabetes, asthma and celiac disease. Likewise, certain Neanderthal inherited genes have proven advantageous or detrimental, such as hair and skin color genes, sleep patterns, and even mood.

Akey has also uncovered genetic signatures that indicate that our human heritage includes organisms we know very little or nothing about. The Denisovans are just one case in point. They coexisted with anatomically modern humans and Neanderthals, an ancestral species of human, and interbred with both before they became extinct. The first evidence of their presence came in 2008 when a finger bone was discovered in Denisova Cave in southern Siberia's isolated Altai Mountains. At first the bone was assumed to be Neanderthal, because there was evidence of these species in the cave. Consequently, she stayed for years before she was examined in a museum cabinet in Leipzig, Germany. But the investigators were dumbfounded when it was. It wasn't a Neanderthal — it was a form of ancient human that was hitherto unknown. "The Denisovans are the first organisms to have been specifically described from their DNA and not from fossil evidence," Akey said.

Since then, continuing genetic work— much of it conducted by Akey and his colleagues — has shown that Denisovans ' closest living relatives are contemporary Melanesians, the inhabitants of Western Pacific's Melanesian islands— areas like New Guinea, Vanuatu, Solomon Islands, and Fiji. These populations bear between 4% and 6% of Denisovan genes, while they carry Neanderthal genes as well.

Events like this illustrate one of the main characteristics of our human race, said Akey, the admixture was a defining feature of our culture. "Admixture has always been around in human history," Akey said. "Populations split up and they come back together." While there is still much debate about the Denisovans, Akey believes that they were most likely closely related to the Neanderthals, perhaps an Eastern version that split off from the latter sometime around 300,000 or 400,000 years ago. Recently, genetic analysis of Denisova Cave fossils has uncovered evidence of a progeny between a Neanderthal woman and a Denisovan male. The daughter was a human who had lived about 90,000 years ago. Akey and other scholars have been able to compile a compelling story of human history by looking at this genetic trail— one that seeks to update our view of early human origins.

Yet, Akey added, there is so much more to learn. "Although we've probably now sequenced 100,000 genomes, and have pretty sophisticated instruments to look at that variability, the more we learn about how to view genetic variation, the more we discover these secret stories in our Genes," he said.

ALTERING DNA AND ITS EFFECTS

DNA is a molecule which is both complex and adaptable. As such, as a result of a phenomenon called evolution, the nucleotide sequences present within it are subject to change. It can prove harmless, beneficial, or even hurtful, based on how a single mutation modifies the genetic makeup of an organism. Occasionally, a mutation can even induce dramatic changes to an affected organism's physiology. To understand the varying effects of mutations properly, of course, it is first necessary to understand what mutations are and how they arise.

Where do mutations occur?

Mutations can be divided into two main categories according to where they occur: somatic mutations and mutations of the germ line. Non-reproductive cells are susceptible to somatic mutations. Most forms of somatic mutations have no obvious effect on a person, because the mutant cells may substitute for the genetically normal body cells. Yet some other mutations can have a major impact on an organism's life and function. For example, somatic mutations causing cell division (especially those enabling cells to uncontrollably divide) are the basis for many forms of cancer.

Mutations of the germ line arise in gametes or in cells that eventually produce gametes. By comparison to somatic mutations, mutations from the germ line are passed on to the progeny of an organism. As a result, the mutation will bear future generations of humans in all their cells (both somatic and germ-line).

What kinds of mutations exist?

Mutations are not only classified by where they occur— they are also often defined by the length of the nucleotide sequences they impact. Changes to short stretches of nucleotides are considered mutations at the gene level as they influence the specific genes that provide guidance for certain functional molecules, including proteins. Changes in these molecules can influence the physical characteristics of an individual to any amount. Mutations which modify longer stretches of DNA (ranging from multiple genes to whole chromosomes) are called chromosome mutations as opposed to gene-level mutations. Such defects are sometimes serious consequences for the species involved. Because gene-level mutations are more frequent than chromosomal mutations, these small modifications to the standard genetic sequence are based on in the following sections.

Base substitution

Base substitutions are the simplest type of mutation at the gene level, and involve swapping one nucleotide to another during DNA replication. For eg, a thymine nucleotide may be substituted in place of a guanine nucleotide, during replication. Only one single nucleotide within a gene sequence is changed with base substitution mutations, so that only one codon is affected.

Although a base substitution affects just one codon in a cell, it can still have a significant impact on the development of proteins. In addition, base substitutions will lead to three separate subcategories of mutations, depending on the nature of the codon transition. The first of these sub-categories consists of missense mutations, in which the altered codon leads to the incorporation of an erroneous amino acid into a protein molecule during translation; the second consists of nonsense mutations, in which the altered codon terminates prematurely the synthesis of a protein molecule; and the third consists of silent mutations, in which the altered codon codes for the same am.

Insertions and deletions

Insertions and deletions are two common forms of mutations which can affect gene level cells. During replication an insertion mutation occurs when an incomplete nucleotide is added to the DNA strand. This can happen when the replicating strand "slips," or wrinkles, which allows to incorporate the extra nucleotide. Strand slippage may also result in mutation deletion. A deletion mutation occurs when a wrinkle appears on the strand of the DNA parent, which eventually causes the replicated strand to lack a nucleotide.

During replication the insertion or deletion of one or more nucleotides may also lead to another type of mutation known as a frameshift mutation. The consequence of a frameshift mutation is complete modification of a protein's amino acid sequence. Such modification happens during translation when ribosomes read the strand of mRNA in terms of codons, or three nucleotide groups. Such classes are called frame comprehension. Thus, if the number of bases removed or inserted into a DNA segment is not a multiple of three (Figure 4a), then the reading frame transcribed to the mRNA will be changed completely (Figure 4b). Consequently, once the mutation is encountered, the ribosome will read the mRNA sequence differently, which may result in the production of a completely different amino acid sequence in the growing polypeptide chain.

Let's use the comparison with terms as codons, and letters within those words as nucleotides, to better understand frameshift mutations. That term has its own distinct meaning, since each codon contains one amino acid. The following sentence consists entirely of three-letter words, each describing a codon of three letters: THE BIG BAD FLY HAD ONE RED EYE AND ONE BLU EYE.

Now, assume a mutation removes the sixth nucleotide, the letter "G" in this case This deletion means letters change, and the remainder of the sentence includes completely new "words": THE BIB ADF LYH ADO NER EDE YEA NDO NEB LUE YE.

This mistake changes the connection of all nucleotides to each codon, which changes every single codon in the sequence effectively. Consequently, the amino acid sequence of the protein is widespreadly evolving. Imagine an example with an RNA sequence, which codes for an amino acid sequence: AUG AAA CUU CGC AGG AUG AUG AUG

The sequence shown in Figure 5 refers to a protein consisting of the following amino acids with the triplet code: Methionine-Lysine-Leucine-Arginine-Arginine-Methionine-Methionine-Methionin

So, assume a mutation takes place during transcription, resulting in the template losing the fourth nucleotide. The nucleotide sequence would now read the following when broken into triplet codons: AUG AAC UUC GCA GGA UGA UGA UG

This set of codons would encrypt the following amino acid sequence: Methionine-Asparagine-Phenylalanine-Alanine-Glycine-STOP-STOP

At that point, each of the stop codons tells the ribosome to end protein synthesis. Consequently, because of the deletion of the fourth nucleotide, the mutant protein is completely different, and it is also shorter due to the appearance of premature stop codon. This mutant protein cannot perform its proper function in the cell.

What causes mutations?

Mutations in cells of all types can arise as a result of a variety of factors, including chance. In fact, some of the above-mentioned mutations result from spontaneous events during replication, and are thus known as spontaneous mutations. One example of a spontaneous mutation is the slippage of the DNA template strand and subsequent insertion of an extra nucleotide; another is the excess flexibility of the DNA strand and subsequent mispairing of the bases.

Environmental exposure to certain chemical substances, ultraviolet radiation or other external factors may also lead to changes in DNA. These genetically modified external agents are called mutagens. Mutagens exposure often leads to alterations in nucleotide molecular structure, ultimately causing DNA sequence substitutions, insertions, and deletions.

What are the consequences of mutations?

Mutations are a cause of genetic diversity in organisms, and they can have widely varying effects on humans, as mentioned earlier. In some cases, mutations prove beneficial for an organism by allowing it to adapt better to environmental factors. In other situations, mutations are harmful to an organism— for example; they may result in increased susceptibility to disease or illness. Mutations are benign in other cases, and do not prove beneficial or harmful to an organism. Therefore it is safe to say that the end consequences of mutations are as complex as the mutation forms themselves.

CONSEQUENCES OF DNA MISINFORMATION

Evidence of DNA is potent but it has limitations. Another drawback applies to misunderstandings about what a DNA match actually means. Matching Evidence from a crime scene to a suspect's DNA isn't an absolute guarantee of the suspect's guilt. Forensic experts instead prefer to speak about probability. For examples, they might make a statement like this: the probability is 1/7,000 that an unknown individual would by accident have the same DNA profile as the evidence. Combine the statistical analysis with other facts, and you can see how prosecutors can deal with a suspect in strong cases.

How the DNA research is presented in movies and television is a contributing factor to widespread misunderstanding. Many lawyers and judges argue that criminal justice is affected by a so-called "CSI effect" The CSI influence shows itself when judges seek DNA testing in situations where it is inappropriate or relies too heavily on DNA evidence to the exclusion of other physical evidence obtained at a crime scene.

More disturbing are cases of DNA fraud— cases where criminals are planting fake DNA samples at a crime scene. In 1992, false DNA evidence was planted in his own body by Canadian surgeon John

Schneeberger, to avoid suspicion in a rape case. Planting fake DNA that someone else obtains is just part of the problem. Scientists at Nucleix, an Israeli firm, recently reported that they could generate a sample of DNA without having any tissue from that human, with access to profiles contained in one of the DNA databases.

Nucleix has developed a tool for separating actual DNA samples from fake ones, with the goal of marketing the product to forensic laboratories. But making such extra precautions to ensure the findings are accurate will only slow down the busy laboratories even more. In reality, backlogs in forensic casework are becoming a serious issue. A study conducted by the Bureau of Justice Statistics showed that more than half a million investigations have been stalled in forensic labs, which suggests that felons and other violent offenders could walk the streets because their DNA evidence is held in a queue waiting for processing.

When progress is made in DNA testing some of these problems may become less serious. But there will likely be other, unforeseen challenges. Next we will look at some of those advances and their implications.

BALANCING AND HEAL BODY'S STRUCTURE

"Structural equilibrium" for your wellbeing is usually considered literally as a good or bad pose, but that's just part of the picture. Structural harmony has a very big influence on your overall picture of health. Because of structural imbalance, you can suffer joint pain, stomach disturbances, "nerve" disorders, easily damaged joints and many other problems.

The body is kept erect and muscles move. The only thing a muscle can do is move two points of attachment closer together; consequently there must be an opposing muscle pulling back for each muscle action. This can be explained clearly by two muscles pushing on an upright post in equal measure. If one muscle gets a nerve impulse that causes it to contract, the other muscle has to relax enough to "carry out" its length so the post can travel. Clearly, if in the nervous system anything goes wrong that does not cause the second muscle to relax, then the contracting muscle cannot move the post over. That simple principle is present when you walk and go about your everyday activities in a very complex manner.

Occasionally something happens in the nervous system which causes the mentioned muscular activity to be unable to function. If a muscle is damaged by contracting or extending beyond its natural tolerance, it will stay in a contract or relaxing state until something is done to return it to normal. Often "everything" is nothing more than the comfort of a good night. If the muscle dysfunction does not return to normal within a reasonable time, care would likely be required.

Many parts of the nervous system function in a similar fashion to the circuit breakers and fuses inside your home. When an organ or muscle is overwhelmed by an injury or action, a protective mechanism occurs that deactivates the organ or muscle for its own protection. In other words, it will blast out the "circuit breaker," thereby preventing the organ or tissue from overloading. The muscle or organ will not function at its optimal level until the nerve center is activated.

Throughout chiropractic, the technique of applied kinesiology will find muscles and nerves that do not operate at their maximum rate and assess the position of the "circuit breaker" nerve; therapy is then used to restore normal function.

The body is kept in place by antagonistic forces pushing against each other in equal measure. Stress occurs at the joint when they don't work equally and it becomes susceptible to injury. It may cause osteoarthritis (the form of arthritis called "wear and tear") to develop over a long period of time at a joint. If a young child has imbalance, the shape of the bones may be altered. This can cause the abnormal bone and joint shape to have a permanent knock-knee or bowleg state. A person who sprains an ankle regularly is usually the result of imbalanced muscles in the lower portion of the leg keeping the ankle in place.

Most nagging low back pains are caused by a change in postural balance due to relaxation of some muscles and contraction of others. Many so-called "clumsy" kids are really victims of muscle dysfunction, creating complicated and uncoordinated movement.

A chronic vertebral or pelvic subluxation is one of the most important involvements in structural imbalance. When there is a chronic subluxation to the vertebral or pelvic. If there is an inconsistency in one of the muscles holding a vertebra or the pelvis in place, after a change the system will revert to an unnatural state-possibly within minutes. Applied kinesiology test helps to find the reversal of these muscle imbalances. Afterwards the correction of subluxation is preserved.

Recurrent vertebral subluxation is most important because it can affect nerves that disrupt control of the tissue, organ, or system supplied by the nerve involved, causing some sort of loss of health.

Your doctor will check several different muscles using applied kinesiology methods to assess the structural equilibrium in your body. Muscles that are low, when the right therapy is administered, should easily return to normal. Because some of the damaged nerves have already been active for a long time, the same region may need to be repaired multiple times; however, if frequent repair is needed, the continued problem is caused by something. The doctor will check until he discovers and removes the exact cause, so that you can live a comfortable, healthy life.

THE EXPERIENCE OF CONSCIOUS INTENTION

Any theory of consciousness is primarily aimed at providing an informative account of what makes the difference between conscious and unconscious mental states. Typically, whether or not a given theory is successful in this regard is measured in terms of its ability to explain what it is to be conscious, for example, of visual, auditory or somatosensory states that are paradigmatically sensitive. And it is often believed, either implicitly or explicitly, that whatever framework is given for such states can be extended safely to fit other mental state forms as well.

Here I dispute this conclusion, as it applies to the philosophy of consciousness in Jesse Prinz's Attended Intermediate-level Representation (AIR). I raise doubts, in particular, as to whether the theory in its present form can account for conscious intentions, largely deriving from a pair of its core obligations. First, the AIR theory has it that "consciousness arises when and only when attentiveness modulates intermediate-level representations. Secondly, Prinz argues that "every consciousness is perceptual" Or put it another way, all conscious systems are sensory states. So the AIR theory poses the following dilemma: either conscious intentions are intermediate-level sensory images that we can attend to, or our intentions are never conscious despite appearances to the contrary. I will present some reasons for being skeptical about the viability of these two options, which together suggest that the theory of AIR does not, as it stands, have the means to explain conscious intentions.

However, before getting to these concerns, it will be useful to clarify what Prinz means by representations of "intermediate-level," "sensory," and "attended." An intermediate-level representation is defined in terms of the degree of specificity of its text, compared to high-level and low-level representations. For example, in perception, high-level states reflect categorical characteristics of objects in an invariant manner, while low-level states represent specific local characteristics of objects such as edges and orientation, and intermediate-level states represent object characteristics such as borders and contours from a particular point of view. When such states are modulated by attention, they are made available for further processing to the working memory, which allows the use of these representations in additional capacities such as verbal reporting and reasoning. Finally, a sensory state for Prinz refers to a state with a representational format specific to a sensory modality, which is itself construed as a dedicated system of inputs.

Considering these conditions, why not simply view conscious thoughts as aided sensory experiences of the intermediate level? Indeed Prinz pursues a parallel strategy to explain how we can have conscious thoughts, even though though thoughts are high-level states themselves. They insists that thoughts are conscious as long as they are "hidden in sensory vessels and have no attributes above their sensory values." In fact, Prinz believes that by creating an intermediate-level sensory awareness of what it means, and by attending to that state, a perception can be "made conscious." Therefore, for example, as I create a visual perception of, say, the Eiffel Tower and the sun shining upon it, my thinking that Paris is magnificent in the spring is aware. Analogously, the AIR hypothesis might potentially accept cognitive thoughts by treating them as states that become conscious as one shapes and attends to a sensory experience sufficiently linked.

It may seem attractive to this proposal but it faces some serious difficulties. For one we often develop conscious thoughts without any sensory imagery that accompanies them. Once I realize that I am out of the milk, I may form an intention to go later to the store without visualizing my future action. Nevertheless, I could announce my purpose and use it to schedule the rest of my day in the interest of further realistic reasoning. On just about every other theory of consciousness, including the AIR theory, only conscious states are accessed and used in this manner. So it seems that I can have a conscious intention without any sensory vehicle being encoded to it.

But perhaps one will not be moved by this concern because, one might insist, even if some of our conscious intentions are not accompanied by visual imagery, they are accompanied by "inner speech," which is properly regarded as a form of verbal imagery, and thus sensory imagery. The inference I consider implausible. Sometimes we deliberately intend to do something without putting the intention into words yet, even in inner speech. But even if one rejects this, Prinz understands the other issue of catching the attitudinal aspect of a conscious purpose through such verbal imagery. It may be possible to make aware of the nature of an intention by linguistic visualization, but we also need a way to explain intentionally planning to do something rather than, say, actively anticipating that we are going to do it, or consciously desiring to do it, which content-wise may appear the same. Verbal language does not achieve this function.

The approach here for Prinz is to refer to feelings to distinguish the perceptions of our conscious mental states in a tactile way. Applying this to the case of ambition, Prinz writes: "If I want my candidate to win, I can feel an anxious expectation, and the thought of success would rejoice, while the thought of loss would lead to waves of panic. I will say that I want a win anytime I encounter any of these fluctuating emotions. But our conscious intentions have no signature emotional profile to which we can appeal to determine that we intend to do something, as opposed to wanting to do it. To be sure, I am not here arguing that motives include or are followed by characteristics of love or motivation— maybe that is real. Nor do I deny that such qualities would be properly interpreted as sensory qualities— maybe that is true, too. Rather, the worry is that whatever sensory affective or motivational qualities they may involve or be accompanied by, it will not be enough to distinguish between an intention to do something and a desire to do it, as a desire will be accompanied by those very same qualities.

Moreover, it is worth emphasizing that even if these concerns were addressed successfully, the present proposal would still not actually explain how an unconscious intention becomes a conscious intent. Any conscious sensory images corresponding to the content of unconscious intentions would be clearly distinguished from those intentions, as the intentions are not sensory images themselves. (This also holds true for Prinz's treatment of conscious thoughts.) But then the unconscious intention itself would still be unaware, and so it's hard to see how this proposal helps with our initial challenge. Yes, the fear applies equally to Prinz's conscious thought record.

Another general strategy that Prinz has at his fingertips, as described, is to assume that motives are always intentional, and instead to maintain that we are in error if we consider ourselves to be intentionally conceived. Nonetheless, Prinz seems to be receptive to this notion, clearly considering the opinion that"... we are not consciously aware of action choices, so free will is an artifact to that degree." We never form conscious intentions before action on this proposed view, but we engage in post-hoc, reconstructive inferences that convince us that we are doing so.

Prinz addresses some experimental work undertaken by as support for this theory. The authors used a paradigm of Libet-styl, asking participants sitting in front of a clock to report when they became aware of their decision to act. They then applied transcranial magnetic stimulation (TMS) either directly after the operation was done or 200 m sec later over the pre-supplementary motor field. The surprising result was that decisions of participants on the TMS trials were moved backwards in time when they first became conscious of choosing to act. In other words, when TMS was applied, they mentioned being mindful of intending to act at an earlier time compared with trials where no TMS was administered, concluding that,"... the presumed initiation of behavior depends, at least in part, on neural activity that happens after the action is performed" (p. 81). Based on these findings, Prinz speculates that,"[for everything we know, conscious decisions[...] can occur after action has taken place and then be wrongly backed up to earlier points in time."

But it's not clear how that would deal with the current issue, because Prinz would still have the challenge of describing what it takes to make a conscious decision after the event. I have already raised concerns about perceptual conditions such as those experiencing intermediate-level sensory systems and it is not clear what other choices the AIR theory has to suggest.

Prinz certainly does not need to be wedded to this version of the reconstructive hypothesis. Instead, he has the option to say that no conscious decision ever comes up, even after the action, just the reconstructive inference. But the results do not support that version of the reconstructive hypothesis. It may be that our timing decisions relating to intentions can be affected by events that occur after the action, but while this may indicate that we are often incorrect precisely when we actually make intentions to act— something that would hardly be surprising given how uncommon these judgments are— it does not provide any support whatsoever for the argument that we are sometimes wrong about whether we are shaping To bring this point home, it is worth pointing out that analogous findings of subjective timing distortions related to the onset of sensory experiences, including Libet's own, do not provide evidence that such experiences do not occur, or that we are sometimes wrong to report that they have occurred. Neither are they needed to provide such evidence. There is a clear difference between a judgment that a mental event occurred at time t and a judgment that there was a mental event at all. And we have no reason to be skeptical about our ability to base the results on the latter type of judgment.

Here, Prinz has a reply at his disposal, for there is one putative source of evidence for the reconstructive hypothesis I have yet to address, and that comes from the work of late psychologist Daniel Wegner. One of the most widely discussed studies of Wegner is his "I Spy," which appears to show that sometimes we can also be confused in thinking that we want an action that we do not intend. This would help to reinforce the argument that we are not only often confused about the nature of our plans, but whether or not we wanted to do something first.

Briefly, in the course of the study, participants sat across a confederate and asked to jointly move a computer mouse — in an "ouija board" type set-up — that controlled a cursor on a nearby computer screen, on which a number of objects were displayed. The participants and the confederate would move the cursor together around the screen and were instructed to stop and rate the extent to which they felt they intended to stop at a scale ranging from 0 to 100 after about 30 s ("0" indicating "I allowed the stop to happen" and "100" indicating "I wanted to stop"). What the participants didn't know is that the confederate was in full control of the entity upon which the cursor paused at some trials. However, when participants heard the target object name over headphones just before those stops, they were more likely to give higher scale ratings. The authors conclude that "the forced stops were interpreted as expected"

But, as many have stressed at this point, the results of the experiment do not support this conclusion — so much so that it is somewhat surprising how often this study is cited as proof of the reconstructive hypothesis. Maybe the strongest objection to this interpretation is that, on average, the participants rated the forced stops barely as more than halfway between being allowed and intended. It strongly suggests that they did not see themselves as actively planning the stops but were unsure, if anything, as to their causal connections to the stops. And this is hardly surprising given the highly ambiguous context they were asked to behave within.

CHAPTER 3

CELLULAR LEVEL

Counting the number of cells in the human body is no easier than counting the number of people in the world, but the estimate accepted is 50 trillion, or roughly 10,000 times the present population of the Earth. Isolated and placed under a microscope, the different cell types— heart, liver, brain, kidney, and so forth — look to the untrained eye rather alike. A cell is essentially a bag filled with a combination of water and moving chemicals, surrounded by an outer membrane, the cell layer. A heart, the nucleus, is at the middle of all but the red blood cells, and contains the closely twisted DNA coils. When you keep a speck of liver tissue on your fingers, it appears like the liver of a calf; you would be hard-pressed to distinguish that it is human in particular. Even a skilled geneticist would detect a difference of only 2 per cent between our DNA and a gorilla. Of the many activities of the liver cell, more than 500 at the latest count, simply by looking at it, you wouldn't have an idea.

One thing is unquestionable, as clouded as the mind-body issue has become: somehow human cells have evolved to a state of formidable intelligence. The number of activities in our bodies being coordinated at any given time is quite literally infinite. Like the

Earth's habitats, our metabolism seems to function in separate compartments that are in fact invisibly linked: feeding, sleeping, communicating, speaking, digesting our food, combating pathogens, purifying our toxin blood, renewing our cells, discarding garbage, voting for Republicans, and much more. Every one of these activities weaves his way into the whole fabric. (Our environment is more complex than most people realize. Animals inhabit our earth, as oblivious of our hugeness as we are of their minuteness. Colonies of mites, for example, spend their entire life cycle in our eyelashes.) Within the vast array of the body, the activities of any single cell—like one of the 15 billion neurons in the brain — fill a good medical document. The volumes devoted to any particular body system, such as the immune system or the nervous system, take up many shelves in a scientific library.

In this ultimate ambiguity, the curing process remains somewhere but is elusive. There is no healing organ in there. Then, how does the body know what to do if it is damaged? Medicine has no easy answer. Any of the processes involved in treating a superficial cut — for example, blood clotting — is incredibly complex, so much so that if the system fails, as it does with hemophiliacs, advanced scientific treatment will lose out to recreate the compromised feature. Drugs that replace the missing clotting factor in the blood can be prescribed by a doctor but these are temporary, artificial and have numerous undesirable side effects. The perfect timing for the movement will be lacking, as will the excellent synchronization of a dozen associated procedures. In example, in a land where everyone else is a blood relative, a man-made substance is an enemy. It can never share the knowledge with which all the rest were born.

The body, we must admit, has its own consciousness. Once this enigmatic dimension of our basic nature is known, the magical essence of curing cancer will vanish. The body of everybody knows how to heal a wound, yet it seems that only a few people have bodies that know how to cure cancer.

Thinking about these well-known facts prompted me to come up with three hypotheses. First of all, this wisdom is embedded in our bodies everywhere. Second, our own inner intelligence is far superior to any one that we can attempt to replace from outside. Third, that intelligence is more important than the body's actual matter, as without it, it would be undirected, formless, and chaotic. Intelligence distinguishes between an architect-designed building and a pile of bricks.

Let's keep our word intelligence concept as simple and practical as possible for the moment. Rather than referring to the intellect of a genius, which may seem both exalted and theoretical, I simply define it as "know-how." However you think about intelligence in the abstract, there is no denying that the individual has to be associated with an enormous fund of know-how.

The intrinsic wisdom of the body is so strong that the doctor is met with a profoundly daunting adversary when it goes awry. For example, each cell in the body is programmed by its DNA to separate at a point, creating two new cells after the mother cell splits in half. This method, like everything else governed by our inner intellect, isn't purely mechanical. In response to its own internal need, a cell divides together with signals produced from the cells around it, the brain, the far-off organs that are "talking" to it via chemical messages. Cell division is a well thought-out and carefully considered decision— except for cancer.

Cancer is mad, anti-social behavior, whereby a single cell reproduces itself unchecked and receives no messages from anywhere except, evidently, its own demented Genes. No-one knows why this happens. It's a good bet that the body itself knows how to reverse the process but it doesn't always work for some reason, which is also unknown to science. It's only a matter of time, once the process starts, before the cancer cells invade a vital organ, crowd the normal cells out and cause death. The cancer cells perish with the rest of the body when the final crisis comes, doomed by their ungoverned self-expansion appetite.

Until now, medicine has not figured out a way to send the cancer cells a message in time to ward off the tragic fate they have created. On the level of intelligence, the chemicals which a doctor may use against cancer are not at all effective. Cancer has a mad genius while drugs are simple-minded. Therefore the oncologist returns to a much more barbaric attack, a kind of poisoning. The anti-cancer drug administered is generally toxic to the whole body, but as cancer cells grow much faster than normal cells, they ingest more poison and die first. The entire strategy is a risk that is calculated. The patient must be fortunate; his doctor must be extremely knowledgeable about chemotherapy dosage and timing, both of which are absolutely vital. Then the cancer can be cured, bringing to the patient's lifetime years of useful life.

Ironically, the therapy may fail because it strips the very intelligence that normally protects the body from disease. Many anti-cancer drugs are extremely harmful to the immune system of the body; they directly suppress the bone marrow that produces our white cells, with devastating effects on the number of white cells in the blood. As the chemotherapy progresses, the patient becomes increasingly susceptible to new forms of cancer, and in a number of cases— up to 30 percent for breast cancer— new cancer appears and the patient dies. Additionally, killing every malignant cell is sometimes not statistically possible. It has been estimated that 10 billion cancer cells may be present in an average cancer patient. When his treatment is successful at 99.99 per cent, there would still be 1 million patients, more than enough to restart.

Cancer cells are not created equal; some are more resistant than others, and thus more difficult to kill. It may be that the destruction of the weaker cells acts as a sort of Darwinian selection, leaving the surviving most fit. Chemotherapy, in that case, will actually promote a more virulent illness than it treats. (Similarly, chronic staphylococcus infections in hospitals are often extremely antibiotic resistant because only the most aggressive bacteria can survive in the sterile environment of the operating rooms and endure the constant onslaught of penicillin injections.) It is possible to conceive of a type of "mega cancer" that may develop from one or two malignant cells.

In any case, the early hope that our generation, widely believed in the 1950s, will scrub out cancer with chemotherapy, has sobered. Now a few tumors are overcome at a time, such as childhood lymphocytic leukemia and some types of Hodgkin's lymphoma, while other big victims, such as lung and brain cancers, become virtually untouchable via chemo.

Maybe these results warn us not so much to do further transplant surgery but to look for new skills as a live, active organ in the brain. The brain was the most frozen part of the body's frozen reconstruction paradigm for all that it was glorified by modern medicine, as it alone could not heal itself. This is a curious assertion, on the face of it. At the moment of conception, all the cells in your body, whether a hair follicle, a nerve, or a heart cell, formed from a double strand of DNA. Everything you can do — think, speak, run, play the violin, or rule a country — builds on an ability programmed into that one molecule that originated. But claiming that a brain cannot repair itself is the same as saying that its DNA has been crippled. Is that a rational assumption? The DNA has definitely chosen to become a brain cell rather than a heart cell, and this means revealing some aspects of its capacity while removing others.

But this is far different from saying that capacity was lacking in the Genome. Nothing in DNA is missing. Every cell in the body holds all the infinite possibilities of DNA all along, from the moment of conception to the moment of death. There is evidence of this in the cloning procedure: theoretically, you can take a cell from the inside of your cheek and produce an identical copy of you, or one million identical copies, given the right conditions. Nature's beauty is that she hasn't opted for one million similar clones; however, only the lowest species consist of the same cells, and most of them are single-celled, like the amoeba. But, at the level of DNA, the difference between an amoeba and a human break down in this sense: the entire amoeba is stored in its little package of DNA, and all of you are contained in yours. So it shouldn't be and shocking that a neuron will spontaneously decide to drop its law of not restoring itself (under conditions we don't quite understand) and suddenly start doing just that. The DNA is not weakened.

The truth of the matter is that the brain is too hard to transform into a model and science deals with models by nature. Models are helpful but they have blind spots built into them, without exception. You will have to see it as a very complex and seemingly contradictory aspect, because non-change is maintained in the middle of dynamic change, to see brain function, or any mechanism within the body, without a blueprint.

CHAPTER 4

MESSENGERS FROM SPACE

Climbing to the Incas stronghold town of Machu Picchu is a difficult task. Someone passes a sixteen-thousand-foot pass in the high Andes, where the oxygen is already weak enough to induce giddiness, and once the city is in sight above the clouds, three thousand stone steps enter the walls. This was Pizarro's final captured refuge when he invaded Peru in 1532. One is shocked to learn that Machu Picchu was linked by foot runners with every village along the two thousand miles of the Incan empire. They were fast-paced messengers with almost superhuman stamina. They ran barefoot every day, walking vast distances — at times the size of two to three Olympic marathons. Some of their tracks started in the Colorado Rockies at the height of a mountain peak and climbed more than a mile.

Such riders, Emperor Atahualpa's eyes and ears must have been the ones that warned him of the advancing Spanish. By trait, when he kidnapped (and later murdered) Atahualpa, Pizarro collected a fortune in ransom. One hopes the rumors are accurate that the most valuable Incan gold has been timely secreted away. (Pizarro, who was remarkably arrogant, even for the conquistador, was himself murdered by jealous enemies in 1541.) When you conceive of the human brain as the fortress of Machu Picchu, it must also have runners to take its orders to the farthest outposts of its empire— in this case, the big toe. Indeed, the actual routes are visible— the central nervous system runs down the spinal column, spreading out on either side at each vertebra in the backbone; these main nerves also divide through millions of tinier paths that interact with each part of the body. In the sixteenth century, the early anatomists saw the main nerves but the nervous system kept a secret. Who were the runners who took the signals from and into the brain?

Many people still think the nerves work electrically, like a telegraph system, because that is what medical texts contended until fifteen years ago. A series of important discoveries, though, began in the 1970s, focusing on a new class of minute chemicals called neurotransmitters. These chemicals, as their name implies, transmit nerve impulses; they act as "communicator molecules" in our bodies, whereby the brain neurons can speak to the rest of the body.

Neurotransmitters are the runners running to and from the brain, expressing our thoughts, wishes, experiences, intuitions, and visions to every organ within us. The subconscious alone is not limited to any of these cases. Furthermore, none of them are simply intellectual, as they can be translated into chemical signals. Neurotransmitters affect each cell's survival. Wherever an idea needs to go, these molecules need to go too, and without them there can be no ideas. Thinking is to exercise brain chemistry, facilitating a chain of body wide reactions. We have already seen that intelligence pervades physiology as know-how— now it has acquired a material basis.

That gives away this chapter's plot but with none of the drama. In fact, no other recent biomedicine event has been as revolutionary as those discoveries. The arrival of neurotransmitters on the scene makes the connection between mind and matter much more fluid and moving than ever before — far similar to the river form. We also help fill the gap which obviously divides mind and body, one of the most profound mysteries that man has faced since he began to consider what he is.

At first, around 1973, only two neurotransmitters seemed to be required, one to stimulate a distant cell like a muscle, and the other to slow down the operation. Two brain chemicals, acetylcholine and norepinephrine, are doing just that; they are the nervous system's' go' and' slow down' cues. At the time, they were considered revolutionary, because they proved that the impulse sent from one nerve cell to the next was in nature not electrical but chemical. The agreed notion of tiny sparks springing from neuron to neuron was made obsolete all at once. But at first the new chemical model kept retaining the basic theory that only two signals were required. Man-made machines work with just this sort of binary transition, and the brain apparently did so.

Then, as molecular biologists began to investigate more deeply around the world, numerous new neurotransmitters cropped up, each with a different molecular structure and apparently a different message to deliver. Many of them were structurally related, being formed as peptides, complex chains of amino acids of the same kind as those that appear in the proteins that make up every cell, including brain cells.

As these discoveries appeared, a great many riddles continued to be answered, directly or indirectly. When you take a sleeping cat, withdraw a tiny portion of its spinal fluid and inject it into an alive cat, the second cat will fall asleep automatically. This is because the brain of a cat biologically allows the body to sleep, with its own secret sleeping potion. The reverse drug, a wake-up signal, must be injected into the spinal column in order for the patient to wake up once again.

In humans, where the same chemical mechanisms work, the body is awakened in the morning not through a rude internal warning, but through a series of synchronized signals, at first mild, then increasingly stronger, that lift us from deep sleep by stages. The entire process requires a gradual transition, from sleep biochemistry to the wakefulness biochemistry, in four to five steps. If this cycle is disrupted, you don't come as fully awake as you should— the biochemistry has been combined in two separate stages. That's why newborn parents, having to get up multiple times in the night, feel like they're never quite safe in the daytime. Alarm clocks also jolt us out of our normal wake-up habits, causing grogginess that can linger throughout the day, until the next round of sleeping-and-waking readjusts the balance of the mind-body.

Here is an example related to this. All camels exhibit an unusual tolerance for high pain levels— they can calmly chew on thorns while being beaten by an irate camel driver with a stick at the same time. Curious researchers examined the brain cells of camels and found that they produce large amounts of a specific biochemical which, if injected into other animals, also causes them to ignore pain. It is now known that tolerance of sleep and pain depends on the precise chemical messengers produced within the brain.

One by one, numerous other roles were linked to common neurotransmitters that once had "all in your brain." Schizophrenics with acute paranoia and delusional delusions often improve dramatically if they are placed on a pump for kidney dialysis, which removes impurities from the blood. As we have seen, brain experts have discovered that there is a neurotransmitter called dopamine in the schizophrenics brains at abnormally high levels. Recent chemical treatment of the condition includes using psychoactive drugs to reduce dopamine; perhaps it is actually removed from the bloodstream by the dialysis machine, or by a similar by-product.

By the mid-1980s more than fifty such neurotransmitters and neuropeptides were identified, just ten years after the original discovery. All fifty can be formed by our neurons on one side of the synapses, and once they reach the synapses on the other side all fifty can be obtained by the receptor sites. This means an unprecedented versatility for cell-to-cell connectivity. The individual neuron was now seen as a message producer, not just saying "yes" or "no," as a computer does. The repertoire of the brain is much broader, containing thousands of variations of different signals, with no end in sight, as new neurotransmitters begin to be found at a rapid rate.

Which kinds of signals do nerve cells exchange with each other? The answer is terrifying, as some segments of our chemical vocabulary appear to be as specific as ordinary speech, while others are highly ambiguous. The pain tolerance, like that of the camel, relies on the class of biochemicals discovered in the 1970s, called endorphins and enkephalins, which serve as natural painkillers for the body. The term endorphin means "internal opioid," and encephalitis "in the bloodstream." And that's their story: they are like a version of morphine that the brain itself produces.

This previously unknown ability to produce internal opiates proved very interesting. The body has already been suspected of having to be able to regulate the sensation of pain. While insistent, it is not always pain that reflects on our consciousness. Of example, strong emotions will overpower the body's pain signals, as when a mother tries to save her child from a burning house or a wounded soldier pushes on, avoiding the pain of his injuries. Under more ordinary circumstances, we will all to some degree withhold our mind from a minor pain— we don't feel a sore throat, for example, when we're chatting to someone of intense interest.

No system had ever compensated for that despite this widespread experience of having the pain threshold rising and falling. Perhaps medication might describe it using these internal painkillers, the endorphins and enkephalins, which can be created at will by any neuron in the body. The general public was told very easily that the brain produces up to two hundred times more opioids than anything you can find on the market, with the additional bonus that our own painkillers seemed to be non-addictive. Maybe a doctor will anesthetize his patients in the future by relaxing any area of their brains, giving Western medicine a medical version of Chinese acupuncture.

Morphine and endorphins both block pain by filling the neuron with a certain receptor and preventing the entry of other chemicals which carry the pain message. There can be no sense of discomfort without these hormones, no matter how much physical pressure there is. Using this model, an endorphin molecule resembles a specific word, the word painkiller. One might imagine that whenever the word pain comes to the attention of the brain, it has the option to send back painkiller as its answer. Unfortunately later work clouded this simple picture.

It was found that endorphin levels in the body do not equate with how much discomfort is being experienced on a one to one basis. Placebos, or placebo medications will prove this. It is often possible to relieve patients who are in pain by receiving a placebo, usually a coated sugar pill, which they are told is a powerful painkiller. Not everyone will respond to this, but they will usually say that their pain has gone down between 30 and 60 per cent. This result has been noted for centuries, called the placebo effect, but it is highly unpredictable. The doctor cannot say which patients will benefit in advance or to what degree.

Why should a completely inert sugar pill first relieve pain, even the stabbing pain from peptic ulcers or traumatic surgery? Endorphins have to keep the key, it was now discovered. A drug called naloxone acts as a chemical morphine antagonist, meaning it has the ability to knock out morphine molecules from a receptor site. The sense of pain immediately comes back as naloxone is applied on top of a painkiller. The same thing will happen, as it turned out, for placebo. Patients whose discomfort had gone away from the sugar pill indicated that after they took naloxone it returned again. This meant that endorphins and morphine would actually be the same substance, with the difference being that one is created by the liver and the other by the opium poppy.

But again it was only a certain number of patients who displayed this effect. For some patients, naloxone made the pain return in full force; for others, the placebo effect still worked out completely; and for others, only a little of the pain returned. Scientists were in a state of heightened frustration, where they are still. Endorphins are definitely internal painkillers but it wasn't the entire solution to discover these new molecules.

Pain studies have now shown that morphine is not chemically identical with endorphins, that endorphins interact in a more complex way than narcotic drugs, and that any form of pain relief treatment— morphine, endorphins, acupuncture, or hypnosis — is highly variable in efficacy. It was also discovered that endorphins cannot be converted into satisfactory pharmaceuticals: if given through injection, our internal painkillers are just as addictive as heroin.

Soon, to all the other neurotransmitters, the same frustrating complications that scientists ran up against with the endorphins and enkephalines. A neuron does not actually receive a signal from a nearby nerve cell and transfer it unnoticed along to the next synapse, it turns out. That is just one of their options. While no one can describe exactly how neurons receive their chemical signals, or how they move them down their own axons or trunks, it is understood that the mechanism has to be very versatile. The nerve cell will change the message along the way, transforming the molecules it got at point A into another at point B. Additionally, the receptor locations at the ends of nerve cells may change themselves to accept various types of messages; the receiving station on the other side of the synapse is similarly sensitive.

Such ambiguity is in effect a strongly motivating state of affairs for our purposes, because it shows that the body cannot be recognized without the missing ingredient of knowledge. Endorphins ' physical structure, or any other neurochemical, is not nearly as important as their know-how — how they choose their locations, what causes them to behave, how they "speak" to the rest of the body in precise synchronization, etc. Mind is superior to matter even amid a genuine chemical revolution. Indeed, it now seems that any neurotransmitter's molecular structure is completely secondary to the ability of the brain to employ it.

Cell biologists had come as a tremendous surprise that neurotransmitters are nothing special as far as molecules go. All of the protein in our bodies is made up of twenty simple amino acid chains, and these chains can be organized further into longer sequences called peptides. Neuropeptides have their own signature which separates them from other peptide chains in the body, but the same plant, our DNA, makes them all. DNA is the root of all the proteins restoring cells, building new ones, removing damaged or faulty bits of genetic code, fixing cuts and bruises, etc.

The DNA has worked out another use for its common raw materials, the amines, amino acids and peptides, without having to invent a new class of chemicals. Once again, what is important is just the ability to make these various products. The molecules themselves are nothing special though their discovery by a molecular biologist may be unique to science.

Where does neurotransmitter capability come from, then? Maybe we should dig at the emotional impact. It's not really the adrenaline molecule, after all, that helps a mom run into a burning building to save her child or an endorphin molecule that prevents her from seeing the fire. Love makes her rush in, and determination of one mind protects her against pain. It just happens that her mind's attributes have found a chemical pathway that the brain can follow to converse with the body.

Now we got to the core of the matter. Mind by any definition is non-material, yet it has devised a way to work with these complicated communicator molecules in partnership. As we have seen, their connection is so similar the mind without such chemicals cannot be transferred into the body. Yet they are not aware of these substances. Or do they?

The whole paradoxical condition was wittily explained many years ago when the eminent British neurologist and Nobel Prize winner Sir John Eccles was invited to attend a group of parapsychologists, who addressed the regular issues of ESP, telepathy, and psychokinesis—the ability to move physical objects with the subconscious. He told his audience if you want to see true psychokinesis then imagine the feats of mind-over-matter done in the brain. It is quite incredible that the mind manages to move the atoms of hydrogen, carbon, oxygen, and the other ions within the cells of the brain with every movement. It would seem that there is nothing more away than an insubstantial idea and the brain's strong gray matter. The whole trick is done in a way without any apparent connection.

Biology has not resolved the complexity of mind-over-matter, but continues to move on to ever more complex chemical structures that function at finer and finer physiological stages. It is still obvious that nobody will ever locate an object, however minute it may be, that nature has called "intelligence." This is all the more apparent as we know that all the matter in our bodies, large or small, has been constructed with intelligence as an integral feature. While known as the body's chemical genius, DNA itself is made largely of the same basic building blocks as the neurotransmitters it creates and controls. DNA is like a brick factory made of bricks, as well. (The great Hungarian mathematician John von Neumann, besides being the inventor of the modern computer, was interested in robotics of all sorts. On paper he once created a genuinely ingenious machine, a robot capable of building robots similar to himself — in other words, a self-reproducing machine. Our Biology has done the same on a large scale, since the human body is nothing more than derivatives. Which smart is sugar? Yet DNA is really only sugar loops, amines and other basic components. To start with, if these aren't "smart," then DNA couldn't become smart simply by putting together more. In keeping with this line of reasoning, why is the carbon or hydrogen atom in the sugar not clever as well? Maybe it is. Because we will see, if there is wisdom in the body, it must come from somewhere, and that there may be somewhere else.

If we follow the next step in the story of the neurotransmitter, we face another quantum leap in complications, but surprisingly, the relationship between mind and matter is actually beginning to clear up. The brain areas that mediate our emotions— the amygdala and the hypothalamus, also known as "the brain's core"— were both shown to be particularly rich in all of the neurotransmitter community substances. It meant that where the mechanisms of thought are concentrated (meaning many neurons are tightly clustered), the chemicals associated with learning will be as well. At this point a rather well-defined distinction also occurred between chemicals that crossed the distance between brain cells and those that traveled down the bloodstream from the brain. (In my field, endocrinology, one of the defining characteristics of a hormone is that it floats through the blood, a process that is generally much slower than the transmission velocity of a nerve cell that has been clocked at 225 miles per hour; a signal sent from the head to the toe takes less than 1/50th of a second.) Researchers at the National Institute of Mental Health found equally abundant receptors at other sites outside of the brain. Neurotransmitter receptors and neuropeptides were discovered on cells in the immune system called monocytes starting in the early 1980s. "Heart" receptors on white blood cells?—The significance of that discovery would be difficult to exaggerate. In the past, the central nervous system alone was believed to relay messages to the body, rather like a complex communication system that connects the brain to all the organs it needed to "chat" to. In this model, the neurons act like telephone lines conveying the impulses of the brain— that's their special role, performed by no other biochemical device.

Now it has been seen that the brain not only sends signals flowing in straight lines down the axons, or trunks, of the neurons; it circulates information easily throughout the entire inner space of the body. Unlike the neurons that are fixed along the nervous system, the immune system's monocytes travel through the bloodstream, giving them free access to any other cell within the body. Equipped with a language to mirror the sophistication of the nervous system, the immune system is evidently sending and receiving similarly varied signals. In reality, if it takes the processing of neuropeptides and neurotransmitters in our brain cells to be happy, sad, reflective, excited, and so on, then the immune cells must also be happy, sad, thoughtful, excited— indeed, they must be able to express the full range of "names" that neurons do. In addition, monocytes can be thought of as circulating neurons.

With this one observation, the Intelligent Cell idea became full-fledged reality. One kind of decentralized intelligence that contained DNA in every cell was already well established. When Watson and Crick mapped the DNA structure in the early 1950s, studies had shown that this amazing, almost infinitely complex molecule contained all the necessary information to create and sustain human life. Yet gene intellect was seen mainly as set, as DNA itself is the body's most secure molecule, and due to this consistency, each of us is able to inherit genetic traits from our parents— blue eyes, curly hair, facial features, and so on — and maintain them intact to pass them on to our offspring.

The know-how borne by the neurotransmitters and neuropeptides embodied something altogether different: the mind's winged, transient, sensitive intelligence. The wonder is that not only the brain, whose function is to think, is making these "intelligent" chemicals, but the immune system, whose primary role is to protect us from disease. This rapid explosion of messenger molecules, from a brain chemist's perspective, adds a new level of sophistication to his research. But the discovery of "floating" intelligence confirms for us the body model as a river. We wanted a material basis to prove that knowledge runs through us all, and we now have it.

Anyone can see that his mind is filled with a disconcerting flood of impressions which are far too amorphous to pin down. Psychology is limited to words as similarly amorphous as the common word stream of consciousness, to explain it. Today brain researchers have found cascades of brain chemicals as if to flood the current of water that you can literally see and reach. But unlike a current, there are no banks in those cascades; they run anywhere and everywhere. For the tiniest fraction of a second they never interrupt this flood either. To turn a brain scientist slows the time to examine the elements of a cascade. The compounds he wants to find are incredibly minute— it took 300,000 sheep brains to produce a single milligram of the compound that the brain uses to activate the thyroid. The cell receptors are not easy to grasp, either. We dance continually on the surface of the cell walls and adjust their form to receive new messages; even one cell can contain hundreds or even thousands of locations, of which only one or two can be studied at a time. In the last fifteen years, science has learned more about brain chemistry than it did in all past history, but we are all still like immigrants trying to learn English from paper scraps found on the street.

No one has yet been able to grasp how the chemical cascade is exactly patterning itself to do all the things that a mind can do. Mind, memory, vision, and all the mind's other daily activities remain a deep mystery with regards to their actual mechanisms. But we now know the body and mind are like parallel universes. Whatever happens in the mental universe has to leave tracks in the physical one.

Brain experts have recently found a way to capture 3-D images of a vision, like a hologram. The procedure, called PET (positron-emission tomography), is performed by injecting glucose into the bloodstream whose carbon molecules have been tagged with radioisotopes. Glucose is the only food in the brain that it uses much more quickly than ordinary tissues. Consequently, when the injected glucose reaches the brain, its carbon marker molecules can be picked out as the brain uses them, and thus pictured on a monitor in three dimensions, much the same way a CAT scan is made. Watching these marker molecules change as the brain thinks, scientists saw that each distinct experience in the mind universe — such as a sense of discomfort or a clear memory — triggers a new chemical pattern in the brain, not just at one location, but at many locations. For every thought, the image looks different, and if one could extend the portrait to be full-length, there's no doubt that the entire body changes at the same time, thanks to the cascades of neurotransmitters and related messenger molecules.

As you see right now, in 3-D, your body is the physical image of what you are thinking. There are several explanations why this incredible truth fails our knowledge. One is that with every thinking the actual shape of the body doesn't drastically change. Even so, thoughts are evidently projecting throughout the body. Literally, from the constant play of their facial expressions we read the minds of other people; without labeling it, we often document the thousand fold movements in body language as a symbol of their moods and attitudes towards us. Films made by sleep labs show that we change position dozens of times during the night, obeying commands from the brain we are unaware of.

Third, we don't see our bodies as predicted emotions because there are many physical changes that cannot be interpreted as triggers for thinking. We include minute changes in cell composition, body temperature, electrical charge, blood pressure, and so on, which are not registered at our concentration. You can however be confident that the body is perfectly fluid to mirror any emotional occurrence. By turning the whole lot anything can move.

The new neurobiology discoveries are making an even stronger case for the alternate mind and body worlds. As researchers looked beyond the nervous system and the immune system, they began finding the same neuropeptides and receptors in other tissues, such as intestines, lungs, liver, and back, for them. There is every hope that they too will be found elsewhere. It means the kidneys can "think," in the sense that they can generate the same neuropeptides that are present in the brain. The receptor sites aren't just fuzzy spots. We are questions that demand answers, presented in chemical universe terminology. If we had the entire vocabulary and not just a few bits, we would very likely find that every cell speaks as fluently as we do.

The questions and answers continue inside of us indefinitely. On its own, a single gland like the thyroid has so much to say to the brain, its fellow endocrine glands, and through them to the whole body, that its cascade of communication affects hundreds of vital functions, such as development, metabolism, and much more. How easily you thought, how tall you are, and, for starters, the measurements of your eyes all depend partly on thyroid advice. So we can safely conclude that by some neat partition set up for our own convenience, consciousness is not limited to the brain. In the inner space the mind is reflected everywhere.

Dr. Candace Pert, head of the brain biochemistry division at the National Institute of Mental Health, one of the most forward-looking and experienced researchers in the field of brain chemistry, points out that it is somewhat subjective to assume that a molecule such as DNA or a neurotransmitter belongs to the body rather than to the mind. DNA is almost as much plain knowledge as it is important. Dr. Pert refers to the whole mind-body system as an "information network," shifting the focus away from the gross level of matter to the subtler level of knowledge.

Is there really any need to separate mind and body at all? Pert tends to use one word in her own works for both— the bodymind. If this term sticks it will mean precisely that a wall is crashing down. Pert still doesn't have all of the medical science behind her, but that can change very fast. Every day it is evident that both mind and body are remarkably similar. Insulin, a hormone which is always associated with the pancreas, is now also considered to be formed by the liver, just as the stomach releases brain chemicals such as transfer on and

CCK.

It shows that our smooth separation of the body into the nervous system, the endocrine system, the digestive system and so forth is only partially correct and may likely be outmoded. It has now been absolutely proven that the same neurochemicals damage the bodymind as a whole. At the neuropeptide level, everything is interconnected; therefore, separating those areas is simply bad science.

A body that can "think" is far from being treated now by the one medicine. As one thing, it knows what's happening to it, not only through the cortex, but there's a receptor as messenger molecules anywhere, which means on every cell. It describes much that had not been understood about medications and their side effects. These medications have a disconcerting number of side effects. I can find page after page under the label for corticosteroids if I check my physician's Desk Guide, which lists comprehensively the medications a doctor can recommend. Cortisone is the most common corticosteroid (or just steroid) but it is widely prescribed for the whole family to combat wounds, asthma, arthritis, postoperative pain, and hundreds of other disorders.

If you weren't familiar with receptor sites, steroids would seem particularly unusual. Let us say I recommend steroids to a woman who has a difficult case of arthritis. The steroids would significantly bring down the swelling in their joints but then a host of odd things could happen. She could start complaining that she was fatigued and depressed. Abnormal fatty deposits could begin to appear beneath her skin, and her blood vessels could become so fragile that she would develop very slow-healing, large bruises. What could be the connection between these totally divergent symptoms?

The answer lies on receptor point. Corticosteroids remove some of the adrenal cortex secretions, which is a yellowish layer at the tip of the adrenal glands. At the same time, the other adrenal hormones are blocked, as are secretions from the pituitary gland found in the brain. The steroid surges in and fills all the receptors throughout the body who are "listening" to a certain message as soon as it is sent. That happens when a receiver gets filled is not a simple action. The cell may in other ways view the adrenal "call," depending on how long the site remains full. The receptor remains filled in indefinitely in this situation. (It is important that other signals are not received, as is the lack of countless contacts with the other endocrine glands.) The cell will experience extreme reactions with one receptor being filled in. By comparison, on a summer night, look at a moth lying under eaves. The fluffy antennae on her back, in a male moth, are simply receptor locations that have spread outside the body. As the sun sets, the moth is looking for a signal from a nearby female moth releasing a special molecule called a pheromone. Moths are small insects, and the amount of pheromones they will carry through the air is infinitesimal compared to the total volume of air and its enormous load of pollen, dust, water and other pheromones that animals of all sorts, including humans, secrete. One would not believe two moths could interact over any distance of any duration.

But when a single molecule of pheromones arrive on the male antenna, its action is changed. He immediately homes in on the female, begins an intricate ceremony of courtship in the air, and continues with the mating act. Biologically speaking, one single molecule is the only thing that causes this complex action.

CHAPTER 5

THE QUANTUM MECHANICAL HUMAN BODY

The concepts in quantum physics remain a total mystery for most people ninety years after they began to emerge. Yet once you understand what neuropeptide discovery means, then understanding the quantum is just one step further. Neuropeptide discovery was so important, as it proved that the body is flexible enough to suit the mind. Events that seem completely unconnected — such as a thought and a bodily reaction — are now seen to be consistent thanks to messenger molecules. The neuropeptide is not a feeling, but it travels through thought and acts as a transition point. Except that the entity in question is the universe, or humanity as a whole, the quantum does exactly the same thing.

To really grasp how the mind pivots on a molecule's turning point we must read the quantum. At the touch of a finger, a neuropeptide bursts into life but from where does it spring? In a hidden process, a transformation of non-matter into matter, a thought of fear and the neurochemical which it turns into are somehow connected.

The same thing happens all over nature except we don't call it thinking. The landscape is not one of solid objects moving around like partners in a dance, following predictable steps, when you get to the level of atoms. Subatomic particles are separated by huge gaps, making each atom empty space more than 99.999 per cent. That refers to hydrogen atoms in the air and carbon atoms in the wood which are made of tables, as well as all the "solid" atoms in our bodies. So all solids, including our bodies, are proportionately as hollow as intergalactic space.

How could these vast stretches of space, filled by specks of matter at far-off intervals, turn into humans? A quantum perspective is required to answer the problem. We enter a vaster reality, spanning from quarks to galaxies, by understanding the quantique. At the same time, it turns out that the behavior of quantum reality is very intimate to us— indeed, the weakest shadow line separates the human body from the cosmic body.

Whenever any mental event is required to find a physical counterpart, it works through the human body's quantum mechanical. That is the secret of how the two worlds of mind and matter became unerringly linked with each other. Mind and body are both saturated through with knowledge, no matter how different they look. Science appears to be suspicious in the face of any argument that wisdom is at work in nature (this is a curious historical anomaly, since each generation before us has embraced some sort of universal order without question). However, if there is nothing to hold things and events together outside ordinary reality, then one is led into a set of impossibilities.

We can see this in the Gravity Theory. Common sense says that two objects separated by empty space should have no connection with each other; they occupy their own "local reality" in the jargon of physics, but the Earth revolves around the sun, gravitationally held in its orbit, even though the two bodies are separated by a 93 million-mile void. Newton was surprised when he learned this breach of social truth and declined to comment on how it was going to happen. Regional history has taken one pounding after the other ever since. Light, radio waves, lasers, and all other electromagnetic forces pass through empty space; matter and antimatter appear to exist in organized universes that have no physical contact; subatomic particles have spins that match each other, and it doesn't matter how far apart the particles are in time and space— their spins and align at opposite ends of the universe.

What this implies is that only at a certain level the common sense idea of local reality is true. As quantum physics explains, the whole of reality is lying deeper. A popular mathematical formula, known as Bell's theorem (after its founder, the Irish physicist John Bell), argues that the truth of the universe must be non-local; in other words, all objects and events in the world are entangled and refer to the changes in state of each other. Bell's theorem was formulated in 1964, but decades earlier, the great English astronomer Sir Arthur Eddington had anticipated interconnectedness by saying, "When the electron vibrates, the universe shakes." Physicists now accept interconnectedness as a rule principle, along with many forms of symmetry that extend across the universe — for example, it is theorized that every black hole may be matt.

Which sort of description will satisfy Bell's criteria for a fully integrated, non-local reality? It would have to be a quantum theory, because if gravity is present everywhere at the same time, if black holes know what white holes are doing, and if a difference of spin in one particle induces an equal but opposite transition immediately in its counterpart somewhere in outer space, it is clear that the information going from one location to another travels faster than the speed of light. In ordinary reality, that is not allowed either by Newton or Einstein.

Contemporary theorists like the British physicist, David Bohm, who worked extensively with the implications of Bell's theorem, had to assume that there is an "invisible field" that holds together all reality, a field that has the property of knowing what is happening everywhere at once. (The invisible term here means not only invisible to the eye but undetectable to any measurement instrument.) Without going deeper into these speculations, one can see that the unseen environment sounds very much like the inherent intellect of DNA, and both behave very much like the subconscious. The mind has the property of holding all of our ideas in place, so to speak, in a silent reservoir where they are organized precisely into concepts and categories.

By naming it "thought," we may be watching nature think through many different channels, one of the most fortunate of which our minds are, because the mind will construct and feel the physical truth at the same time. It may seem completely rational to observe a quantum phenomenon in the context of light waves, but what if quantum truth was just as apparent in our own feelings, impulses and desires? Eddington once expressed flatly his assumption as a scientist that "the world's stuff is mind-stuff." Thus the quantum mechanical system, as knowledge creation, has a possible position in non-local reality.

The benefit of such a simple image is that knowledge is basic; the complications arise when one manages to track down the mind-body system's incredibly complex mechanism. A psychopath and a poet's brain-wave signals appear the same on a EEG paper roll as they come off the electroencephalograph, no matter how advanced the study is. Thinking about the thousands of hours it would take to objectively explain the chemical effects of the daily life of one person, a neuroscientist friend of mine commented, "You have to say that nature is intelligent because it is too difficult to name anything else." He could have said "too easy" just as easily. In ancient India, intelligence was supposed to exist everywhere; it was called Brahman, for "big" from the Sanskrit word, and it was just like an invisible champ. A proverb from thousands of years ago suggests that a man who didn't find Brahman is like a hungry fish who didn't find water.

Our entire physiology can be transformed as fast as a neuropeptide, an integral part of the mechanical body of the quantum. The fluid quality of life is normal to us because we can change like quicksilver. The human body is a river of electrons, the mind is a river of consciousness and it's a river of knowledge that binds them together.

There is much more to be said about the mechanical quantum body. I can't think of anything more we need to know. Medicine today wants to make the leap beyond its current dilemmas, but the will has turned into waiting. As a research physician in the United States, a fellow student from my medical school days in New Delhi has grown meteorically to become a professor at Harvard Medical School before he turned 45. We were alone in a Boston restaurant recently after dinner and he discussed the future. "All the top researchers gathered privately in Congress," he said glumly, "and we concluded that no new disease would be treated by the year 2010, and there would be no advance in discovering AIDS." It might be impeccable science, but from the quantum viewpoint this makes no sense. In the realm of? We are all expert navigators Zone, where science is groping with one slight light. Suggests that not a solution? The mysterious breakdowns of the body's intelligence that occur in cancer and AIDS can all be traceable to a single distortion— a wrong detour into the intelligence's hidden regions of DNA. To see how the problem with the mind-body can be solved, we need to take a closer look at these detours and their invisible origin.

CHAPTER 6

THE QUANTUM BODY IS MORE THAN THE PHYSICAL

No one's ever going to see the artificial quantum body. That will be a problem for many people. Not only scientists but we are all comfortable with things that we can see and touch. Modern medicine's history consists largely of tracking down solid objects that cause disease, though nearly all of them live in the realm of the invisible, beyond anything that the naked eye can perceive.

A canny researcher in fourteenth-century Europe might have conjectured that a rat in the house contended that there was a danger of bubonic plague (probably rats were so prevalent that the correlation was never made); seeing a flea on the rat's pelt brings you closer to the real cause, but only when you study the rat's blood under a microscope and discover the bacterium Pasteurella pestis can you really have one?

What would be a bacterium, without a microscope? Something that is invisible to the eye and yet as wide as the planet as it touches any place on Earth, including the poles. It would come and go like smoke, entering the tightest locked doors and windows— if you trusted only in the senses, such an organism's capacity to be there and at the same time everywhere would appear incredible. The quantum world, in fact, is yet another step down on the invisibility scale. Unlike the tiniest bacteria or viruses, you can never see a single photon, electron or any other entity in the quantum world using any expansion of sight and contact. We are really everywhere and at the same time none at all.

Until very recently this fact scarcely affected medicine, because the smallest virus is still several million times larger than an elementary particle. The germs are also quite elastic in time and space, while the quantum phenomena blink unpredictably into and out of existence. If Pasteurella pestislurks in your blood, it's there, totally and certainly, unlike the ghostly mesons that leave brief highlights on a photographic plate for a few millionths of a second, only to disappear out of material existence, and most unlike the neutrino that can travel undetected through the whole Planet as if nothing was standing in the way.

Until 1987, when a French immunologist, Jacques Benveniste, performed an experiment that is outrageous to all nonquantum views of the world, the vast difference in scale between medicine and quantum physics kept the two sciences on separate ground safe. The experiment started innocuously on the soil. Dr. Benveniste took a common antibody called IgE (standing for type E immunoglobulin) and exposed it to some white blood cells called basophils. What happens when these two interact–the IgE antibody clamps and waits firmly on specific receptor sites–is well known. What it is waiting for is an invading molecule floating in the bloodstream, against which it needs to be defended. The invader in this case is not a germ but an antigen, a material which causes allergies.

If you're allergic to bee sting, the bee venom molecules wouldn't be longer than a few seconds in your bloodstream before they activated the IgE antibody. It would in turn set off a complex chain reaction in the cell that would throw the body's allergic response into high gear; the basophil would release a chemical called histamine that causes the typical allergy attack swelling, redness, itching, and shortness of breath. The mystery in allergies is that the antigens, the offending substances that enter the body, are generally harmless— wool, pollen, dust— and yet they are treated as the deadliest enemy by the immune systems. Allergies were thoroughly studied at the molecular level to find their cause, and one of the outcomes is a firm grasp of IgE.

That sets the stage for a dramatic experiment by Dr. Benveniste. He took some human blood serum full of white cells and IgE, and combined it with a formula made from the blood of goat that was sure to cause histamine production. This second solution contained an anti-IgE antibody, representing venom for bee, pollen, or other antigens. When the IgE and the anti-IgE hit, the test tube reaction went off exactly as it would in a person with a bad allergy and it produced large amounts of histamine.

Benveniste then distilled and applied the anti-IgE tenfold again — still the same reaction. He began to dilute, time after time, and as before, about half of the IgE started to respond (40 to 60 per cent). This was extremely surprising, because he was just past the limit that chemically active solvent should be. He decided to further dilute the anti-IgE, making it one hundred times weaker each time, until he knew there was no anti-IgE at all. His last dilution included 1 part of an antibody to 10120 parts of water; this amount would be represented as 10, if printed, followed by 120 zeroes. Using a constant dubbed the amount of Avogadro, he mathematically proved that it was unlikely for the water to produce a single antibody molecule. When he added this "solution," now merely distilled water, he set off the histamine reaction with the same power as before. (The classic Humphrey Bogart movie, To Have and Have Not, features the quirky line, "Have you ever been stung by a dead bee?" In this situation, the bee is also invisible.) Although its conclusion was an impossibility, Benveniste duplicated it seventy times, and challenged other research teams to replicate it in Israel, Canada and Italy — all ended up with the same result. They also found that an antigen that's not there would activate the immune system. Benveniste has discovered the spirit of history in our terms — he himself speculates that water contains the spectral traces of the molecules that once stood in it. His observations were published reticently in the June 1988 edition of the prestigious British journal Nature. His editors have openly stated their repugnance to the outcome, correctly arguing that "there is no physical basis" for it. The human white cells were behaving as if they were being targeted from everywhere by the anti-IgE when it was in fact zero.

Medicine is hesitant to step through the quantum door although it is obviously opened by this experiment. Benveniste was widely held to be lending credence to homeopathy methods, a medical system invented two hundred years ago by a German physicist, Samuel

Hahnemann, and still popular across Europe. The term homeopathy comes from two Greek roots meaning "similar suffering;" this points to the fundamental homeopathic principle that "like treating like." Homeopathy approaches all diseases using Benveniste's method: the patient takes tiny amounts of antagonistic substances to build up immunity or drive out a disease if it is already present.

It suggests the homeopathic theory is at work while conventional medicine administers a smallpox vaccine— the dead virus in the vaccine triggers anti-smallpox antibodies in the body. (This way of treating smallpox dates back to ancient China, where physicians learned how to take scabs from the sores of victims of smallpox and put them on small cuts in the bodies of those they wanted to protect from the disease.) Unlike vaccines, though, homeopathy is based on symptoms rather than on real disease-causing bacteria.

The homeopath uses an elaborate system of poisons and toxic herbs that mimic the symptoms of true disease, giving the body a taste of what it wants to cure. For example, ground-up Nux vomica seeds containing strychnine would be administered to counteract chronic fatigue and irritability, because these symptoms themselves are produced. In reality, Benveniste's experiment did not endorse homeopathic theory as a whole but just one corner of it, by demonstrating that the body would respond to a foreign substance's microdose. The bulk of homeopathy is unequivocal. (The principle of "like treatments" is accepted in Ayurveda, and even extended to say that every part of the body is matched by herbs, minerals, and even colors and sounds that can be used to treat it. However, Ayurveda does not follow the homeopathic logic of making the body sick to make it healthy.)

THE HEALING PATH TO SUPRAMENTAL INTELLIGENCE

The Triple Transformation The Indian seer explains three consecutive stages of this transformation for those who follow the journey of personal transformation (i.e. yoga), Sri Aurobindo, the intellectual, the spiritual, and the supramental.

One passes from the outer surface consciousness to the inner consciousness in the first step of the Triple Transformation; the mental subconscious, the subliminal beyond, until one meets the real spirit, that is, the true psychic consciousness. At the spiritual one has separated from the ego-consciousness, one is able to understand and control the limits of one's physical, essential, and emotional nature, and one is brought into contact with celestial, fundamental powers and realities. This is the Transformation of the Psychic.

At a further point one grows further in one's being towards other realms of consciousness, like Further Consciousness, Illuminated Thought, and Intuitive Mind. It is an access to the world above, an ascent to the upper of one's lower consciousness and the descent to the bottom of the latter. This is the transformation of the Spirit, beyond the Psychic Transformation. Beyond that there is still the Supramental transition, where one rises to the level of the

Supermind, for a radical transformation of the being out of the confusion that is the basis of our being, and into a modern working that transcends the emotional, essential, and physical dimensions. One could be the Supramental Being. These three types are the Triple Transformation which would happen in succession.

When one opens up to the Supramental Consciousness, that is, the Force, one lives, one experiences all its advantages. It can change nature, cause falsehoods to evaporate, generate information where misinformation resides, correct problems, give the full truth and awareness, expose solutions that simultaneously provide harmony for multiple parties, require infinite possibilities, possibilities that can transcend space and time, etc.

Below we list a number of possible ways this Supramental, evolutionary being could work in the world.

Nature of the Supramentalized Individual

GENERAL

As the metaphysical transition has to call for completion into the divine, so the supernatural has to call the Supramental to fulfill it.

The last transformation completes the soul's journey through the Ignorance. This Reality Consciousness has to fall into ready Nature, allowing for the liberation of the supramental concept in her.

ONENESS, UNITY, FLUIDITY

The individual of the Suprament would see everything in its oneness. In all things he will recognize this unity; in the greatest multiplicity and complexity of things; in the individuality of each person and thing; even in what seems as inconsistencies or contradictory components. Therefore he sees everything in their proper relationship to each other and to the whole, the One.

Nature is a life of necessary, natural and intrinsic peace and equilibrium It would be one in its nature the inner, what is within, and the outside, what is outside of it in the universe. He will experience and see this inner-outer interaction of life on an ongoing basis, thus supplying him with the absolute efficiencies of life; causing the limitless possibilities to emerge when traditionally there was only finite possibility.

From the standpoint of unity one sees everything (including contradictions, dualities)

EXAMPLE: One is involved in a project involving a number of companies, each seemingly going through their own development and problems. Through his involvement in the project, through the unfolding of the project, he is able to see all the forces at work (positive and negative) in the midst of all the companies, the individuals he associates with and his own work and development. He knows that in oneness, everything is related, and acts accordingly.

To all the surprises and challenges there would be a calm and deep dignity of mind. One is in a state of peace and equality, unmoved by any circumstances of both positive and negative extremes.

One senses the world's unity in its infinite diversity and complexity.

One sees the unfolding of one's life as one with the unfolding of the spiritual unfolding of the universe Life around one becomes self-possessed, spontaneous, and plastic One sees the unfolding and growth of one's life as one with the unfolding and growth of one's soul, that is, one with the circumstances of one's life.

Another behaves of genuine compassion for everything in the universe All other human creatures would be perceived as his own; would be treated as his own self. Their feelings are his own. His being would spread to others. In everything, including others, he would experience the spirit, which would be the connecting factor that creates the feeling of oneness.

Someone sees the point of view of the other person by his quiet influence He would be one with the energies and influences within his individual self; of the forces in the climate, the culture, the civilization, the earth and the cosmos. He will witness the interrelationship of all powers across the universe, both visible and spiritual. He would also know that he was serving not only his own purpose through his new status, but the purpose of the universe's existence.

A mystical or gnostic social life will inevitably arise from many people who have this supra-mental consciousness. Through regular experiences of cause and effect, space and time, objectivity and subjectivity, we no longer perceive the world. All those mental perceptions are transcended in our new perception and experience of the world.

We become mindful of how the world around us relates to our own state of being (Inner-Outer Correspondence), and know what step (inner and outer) to take to harmonize the two in life.

One has the triple-time vision; knowledge of past, present and future at the same time.

One experiences the Infinite in the finite, the Timeless in time; the One in the many (e.g. in one's own self all selves, and vice versa).

Whereas mind and spiritualized mind view the object of perception, inquiry, understanding as outside one's self, this object is inside one's self in Supermind. Therefore it does not require an object of perception, since the object is a part of itself. One is actually the very object itself. (Just as the Supermind created the world out of nothing, i.e. self-conceived, objectivized a universe of forms out of the Absolute, so can the supramental individual apprehend knowledge, i.e. self-conceiving knowledge, inquiry, perception from within themselves.

ACTION, ACCOMPLISHMENT

One does not pursue the fruit or result; the pleasure of being and doing is linked to the Spirit Instead of being a mere marionette of nature and its will, the person will obey his inner transcendent intent.

There is no need to exercise mental control to achieve results in life

One has full access to the Supramental Force that can accomplish anything at any time, even instantly matching One's own actions, initiatives, etc. with parallel movements all over the world.

EXAMPLE: A person uses the spiritual power inside him to lift the organization he leads to far greater success point. In another part of the world, unexpectedly a multinational organization referring to its own organization has a huge leap in its power and progress.

We become mindful of how the world around us relates to our own state of being (Inner-Outer Correspondence), and know what measure (inner and outer) to take to harmonize the two in life.

By understanding the forces that evoke positive responses from life, we create infinite fulfillment. Through opening up to the Force, we induce these from inside, to evoke the most positive life responses that emanate from the behavior of the Force on the causal plane. The normal definitions of cause and effect, space and time, and subjectivity and objectivity contradict the life responses that exist.

One works not for the strength, happiness, pleasure of the mental and essential ego, but for the Divine in ourselves, in all, in the universe, and appearance instead of the Divine presence, Light, Strength, Happiness, Delight, and Beauty One can produce results in the world as much from the inner being, i.e. from within ourselves, as through our outer actions and experiences. We can create the world from within.

He continuously evokes positive responses to life, allowing him to achieve the level of the normal human being at 1000 times or more. Even 1000 times in a single moment. Thanks to his total consistency and fundamental awareness at any time, he knows exactly what step to take, making for massive immediate and ample outcomes. One's ability to act is balanced by a true knowledge of what is to be desired; and there is the power to make that knowledge work.

He understands the creation process which allowed the Divine to emerge from the universe. As a consequence, he knows how to apply this method in his own life, unlocking life's infinite potential. He achieves this God-power in his own life because he is fully conscious of the process's phases. He is also fully aware of other such cycles of general.

One is constantly opening up to the Power to succeed on infinitely higher rates of existence.

One understands and uses the evidence that to produce a response, one does not need something. Just as the universe emanated from (physical) nothing, so can life emanate from nothing (e.g., you don't really have to work over time to produce results, products don't need materials, etc.). The Supramentalized Person is in touch with and works from Within, delivering endless accomplishment from Nothing through this infinite divine capacity.

The subsequent actions in the Supramental consciousness do not seem to replicate in consistency and character. (This parallels the act of consecration which attracts positive responses in life which seem to be one of a sort, special, unrepeatable.)

DIVINE FOCUS

His life would be one with the soul and the divine and transcendental Soul. His actions were to originate from and obey the divine governance of Nature by the Supreme Self and Spirit. In every core of his mind, in every pulse of his life-force, in every cell of his body he can feel the Divine's power. The acts which he takes (or withheld) would be based on the Divine Will Reality.

He feels that the Divine is his true self and the basis and member to his divine identity. One views the unfolding of his life as one with the emergence of the metaphysical development of the world. One perceives that the universe's intent and fate, which is the spiritualization of the cosmos through the individual's creation, will become not only himself.

One does not act for the power, satisfaction, enjoyment of the mental and vital ego, but for the Divine in oneself, in all, in the world, and the emergence instead of the Divine presence, Light, Power, Love, Delight, and Beauty One would feel the Divine's presence in every part of one's being; one's consciousness, one's life-force, in every cell of one's body, one's whole way of being, one's whole way of thinking, living, one's whole being.

Most precisely, the Supramental and Supramental action is the element of the Supreme that governs all of its creation, nature, and acts. One uses the divine, Supramental Power in one's life to accomplish, eradicate tension, happiness, and salvation.

Ego reaches a point where the arduous task of dissolving itself through spiritual discipline will begin

PHYSICAL, VITAL, MENTAL INTEGRATION

The outer mentality and the nervous being and body would be controlled. One would institute and maintain a right physical perception of things, a right relationship and reaction to objects and energies, a right rhythm of mind and nerve.

DELIGHT OF EXISTENCE

He'd be living in an ecstatic state of happiness, joy and bliss. He would experience a great delight in being at every moment, in every effort, in every encounter with others and in every connection with his environment, in every action that he takes.

Because of the divine virtues within himself, he will feel the continual happiness of life and share the joy of the nature of others. There would be an extreme pleasure in being; in the heart a pride of universal love, unity, compassion, and the joy of being; in the will and vital parts of perceiving and seeing the One everywhere; in the body an ecstasy of harmony and bliss that flows from the spirit.

AWARENESS & KNOWLEDGE

He would have a full knowledge of himself, an essential knowledge. This fundamental awareness will extend to all things, all persons, all times, all scenarios and all situations. He would have the basic, absolute, complete knowledge of what the scenario, condition, or occurrence entails, and what are, if any, the multitude of potential courses of action. He would have the full will to see it through as necessary and he would take the exact right course of action with that energizing him. Thus knowledge, will and outcome of action are fused together in a unity and unity that allows for an integral solution. This allows for the greatest efficiency of life, which is the ability to create the greatest result in the shortest period of time with the least effort.

Direct connection (i.e. is one with) an entity that is part of itself While Intuitive Brain (down to ordinary thought) considers the object as outside, the object is inside in Supermind, and does not need the source of interpretation because the object is part of itself.

One becomes aware of the one truth underlying all things There would be a clearer sense of the truth of oneself and things, and a more enlightened approach to opportunities and difficulties of existence There would be a transcendence of the rigid ways of seeing things in the mentality, its perceptions, its attachment to a fixed set of principles, systems and patterns of life

Evolution in one's life becomes a graded progression from lesser light to greater light One's existence is no longer ideational; i.e. a life based on the knowledge and perception of things. Instead one simply needs to be One has a clear and intrinsic sense of the reality of one's being and one's fundamental understanding of the stuff has the truth of things.

Whereas Intuitive Mind (down to ordinary thinking) sees the object as outside, the object is inside in Supermind, and does not require the object of perception because the object is a part of itself.

One is mindful of other realms of being; and understanding of their energies and influences; (e.g., things in the universe will be seen not only in their visible dimension, but in everything that is hidden and that is actually unfolding) One has a triple-time view, continuous knowledge of history, present and future (There are countless examples that prove that the supramental force's intervention will change the past.

We experience life in such a way that our normal perceptions of cause and effect, space and time, are defiant. For instance, we can change an attitude or perception, or take action that attracts an instant positive response from life (this defies our normal perception of cause and effect; subjectivity and objectivity; time and space). Or a person might believe that a few minutes have passed and an hour has passed; or have the impression that an hour has passed and that only a few minutes have passed (this defies our usual perception of time). One constantly opens up to the Force to attain the fundamental reality, experience, and understanding of the matter.

We are aware of how the reality around us corresponds to our own state of being (Inner-Outer Correspondence), and know what action (inner and outer) to take to harmonize the two in life.

Through knowing the energies that elicit positive responses from creation, we create eternal fulfillment. Through opening to the Light, we enable from within to evoke the most positive responses to creation, which emanate from the behavior of the Spirit on the causal plane.

THE PHYSICAL BEING

The mind would be changed because he understands all objects in their entirety, and has the source of understanding inside him. The knowledge would be he. His relationships with others would be of love and oneness. The body of this individual would be getting great perfection. He could live as long as he wishes; he would be freed from all suffering; and all the pains, injuries, illnesses and other sufferings would be a thing of the past. We would see a dramatic change in his body functions, shape and the possibility of living as long as he wants.

There will be a development that will affect the human being's spiritualization, salvation, and fulfillment; including an evolution of the length of the body, wellbeing, physical beauty, physical joy, freedom from misery, feeling at peace, etc.

There can be a regeneration of the internal senses of one's physical nature There is a divine joy running through the body It has been proposed that the physical body must gradually adapt for the gnostic person. The physical form, for example, may evolve toward a more neutral development, rather than being decidedly male and female. (Even now, the human male develops more grace, subtlety, and flexibility, while the female human gains strength and stamina.) Our organs may also evolve, including the gradual disappearance of the digestive system, the procreative system, and the respiratory system of the lungs.

There may be a means of seeing even without the closed eyes, or listening without using the ears. Many of these functions can gradually shift toward an inner understanding and experience from the outer instrument, organ.

Some have had a vision of a tall, slim individual with little or no breast, neither male nor female, very slim at waist. The transformation and even the possibility of eliminating the current bodily functioning such as breathing, digestion, would exist. This would imply that this future being would be unnecessary for the corresponding physical organs (lungs, digestion, etc.) (Note: A physical transformation is likely to occur after the other changes have happened. The last thing to change is the physical transformation.) People continue to radiate inner glow and illumination.

The human mind and brain may be reduced or eliminated or radically altered as we would be able to perceive the universe specifically without the involvement of the process of thought, of feeling, of the intellectual function.

One begins to develop an inner capacity to experience hearing, seeing and other senses. One can rely less on the external organs (eyes, ears) and experience the world within oneself. One is capable of perceiving the outer world not with the outer senses but with an inner vision and perception more developed.

One uses the Force to overcome our bodies ' current limitations (i.e., lack of flexibility, inertia tendency, disease propensity, even death inevitability).

In the Supramental universe, the more alive one is, and the more the individual has the will over the material in connection with the truth of things. The will acts directly within the substance, and the substance is will-obedient. One possibility, for example, is when you want to move from one place to another, your will is sufficient to carry you without any vehicle or artificial means being necessary. The will of a human has the power to transform matter as it pleases, such as the power to overcome illness. As one likes one can change matter.

One no longer legitimizes the world's (old mental) material rules, including the corporate laws (its needs, health, diet, etc.). When all these things which seem so real vanish in the new consciousness. One no longer lives these expectations, such that we in this material plane will construct infinite miracles.

Awareness in the Body Learns, is converted immediately by Force The individual's structure becomes body, essential, awareness, and spirit. Body is the lowest, and the highest is the Soul. Today we use mind instrumentation when we want the body to learn a new skill–driving, typing, learning a new language etc. The mind first of all learns what the body needs to learn. The learning is then passed on to the body through training through the knowledge and understanding of the mind.

We can therefore infer that if the mind were not open, the body would never know to the full. Sri Aurobindo and The Mother, however, brought a new perspective; that the body should actually discover that its own centre of consciousness is within the body itself. Then the body is able to receive within itself directly through the mind core instead of accessing through the mind. This is an infinitely greater experience. Thus the body is able to learn and be transformed (e.g., healing, infinite life, new organs, changes in cell constituents, etc.) directly from the Force through its mental center, rather than having to go through the mind and vital centers of the being.

OTHER POINTS

Sri Aurobindo says that Being (the Many) manifests from Non-Being (the One), and that both Being and Non-Being are expressions of something greater and inclusive of the two, which he calls the Absolute. Mind can see either Being or Non-being; only the Absolute can be known by the Supermind. He says realizing this truth will carry the power of creation.

Supramental Human Behavior— When one opens to the Supramental Consciousness, that is, the Power, one lives, and enjoys all its rewards. It can transform nature, enable falsehoods to evaporate, create knowledge where ignorance exists, correct problems, give the full truth and knowledge, reveal solutions that simultaneously create unity for multiple parties, allow infinite possibilities, possibilities that can transcend space and time, etc.

The Supramental Individual, Life— The supramental individual will harmonize his individual self with the spiritual self, his individual will, and the spiritual will. He will have an integral knowledge, a light-out of-light revelation. There will be a vast peace and a profound joy in him. He is going to live a life that reconciles freedom and order, between self-expression, that is one's own truth, and the universal truth of things. These are but a few of the ways supramental being would work. It will be the physical aspects which last to shift in the individual's Supramental transformation. That is to say, its outer form, its sound, its internal organs, etc. The Supramental being's ultimate physical capacity is the ability of the individual to live as long as that individual wants.

Ways of Supramental Consciousness Enter Individual— The descent of the Supramental Force from the Supermind plane may come into the individual as Peace, Silence, Light, Power, Knowledge, Ananda, and in other ways. Everything can be learned by the patient, and used to help the person transform.

Transition of the body accompanied by Eternal Life Based on Will— When the transition of the body becomes complete (it will come after the transformation of the other aspects of the being first, including physical, neurological, and mental), the likelihood of the end of being submitted to death will be present. That is to say, people can live as long as they want.

Knowing Beyond Awareness Supramental Consciousness— Only if one has the Supramental Consciousness can one fully comprehend the Divine's structure and workings. Only so much can the Brain perceive and comprehend which is nothing compared to the other. (So only as one grows higher in consciousness, beyond the mind, up to the Supermind can one truly understand and feel the teachings of Sri Aurobindo, including The Eternal Life) Understanding Which Includes Supramental Perception— Beyond the mind's understanding is the reality that the universe is a whole, God, the Divine is indivisible, Life is total, and all are Absolute in being subjective. Only by getting the Supramental vision can that man know.

Supermind gave us the eternal, the timeless, and the spaceless; the limitless potential in the finite. (Translating as infinite potential, achievement, opportunities, happiness, pleasure, grace, wisdom, greatness, etc.) The intervention of the Supramental Force will change past causality to create a new current (e.g. consecration of the source of a disease deliberately identified as chronic or lethal has, on many occasions, been allowed by a practitioner to rediagnose that the condition does not occur). That which seems to be at odds with Supermind is part of a peace. In its harmony and wholeness it sees all such things through due relation to each other. (It sees unity and equilibrium in that which is separated in spirit. There is no mistake as in thought.) Supermind comprehends all things in being and eternal self-consciousness, abstract, immutable, spaceless, hence it comprehends all objects in fluid awareness and rules their rational self-embodiment in space and time. (This is a powerful statement of how because Supermind knows the forces in Being it knows them in becoming.) Supermind sees all the possibilities of Space and Time that Mind cannot understand, without the mistake, groping, and uncertainty of mind. It perceives each capacity in its own power, necessary need, right relationships with others.

Knower, knowledge, in Supermind intelligence is one.

Supermind is the intermediate connection between Existence-Consciousness-Bliss and Mind that can explain each other and establish a relationship between them that will enable us to realize the one Existence, Consciousness, Delight in the mold of mind, life, and body.

WORKING MULTI-DIMENSIONALLY APPLIED KINESIOLOGY (AK) OR MUSCLE TESTING TECHNIQUES

What is muscle testing?

Applied kinesiology (AK) or manual muscle testing (MMT) is also known as muscle testing. It is an alternative method of medicine which claims to effectively diagnose physiological, muscular, chemical and mental illnesses.

Applied kinesiology is not a part of kinesiology , which is the study of the human body's movement.

The basic idea underlying AK is similar to one of Sir Isaac Newton's Laws of Motion, which says, "There is an equal and opposite reaction for every movement of nature." Applied kinesiology takes this principle and applies it to the human body. This ensures that any internal problems you may encounter would be followed by a similar weakness in the body.

Following this thought process, a muscle test should be performed to diagnose any underlying medical condition. Muscle testing done in applied kinesiology differs from standard muscle orthopedic testing.

Here's an example: you've done a muscle test and your bicep is deemed "bad." A person performing the muscle test with a traditional medicine view may suggest working out more at the gym with your biceps.

A person who follows the principles of applied kinesiology may conclude that you have this disability because of an underlying spleen problem.

A brief history of applied kinesiology

The applied kinesiology began in 1964 as a system of muscle testing and therapy with George Goodheart Jr.

Many years later, a group of chiropractors, in a study conducted by Ray Hyman, wanted to show that they could tell the difference between subjects given good sugar (fructose) and poor sugar (glucose).

A drop of sugar water had been dropped on the tongue of a test subject. Then, they measured the strength of the arms of each test subject. The chiropractors expected they could recognize which subject had been given bad sugar based on weakened muscles. Several unsuccessful attempts later, though, they put the study to an end.

More recently these ideas have been refuted and defined in terms of medical disorders and their causes or therapies as "not conforming to scientific fact."

Who practices applied kinesiology?

Applied kinesiology was used by 43 per cent of chiropractic offices in the United States in a 1998 survey conducted by the National Board of Chiropractic Examiners (NBCE). Although most of the practitioners in the survey were chiropractors, there were nutritionists, naturopathic doctors, and massage and physical therapists in the occupations as well.

The Nambudripad Allergy Elimination Technique (NAET) currently promotes the use of applied kinesiology in the management of allergies and other sensitivities.

However, the results of a study conducted in 2001 using muscle tests as an allergy test for wasp venom state that diagnosing allergies is no more helpful than random guessing.

CONNECTING MEDITATION WITH POSITIVE CHANGES IN THE BRAIN

Vital signs are seen to improve, and with much greater accuracy, various impacts on brain function can be detected. Skeptics were completely pushed out of the debate on these topics, but not on the notion of unbounded consciousness. Recognition of a fourth state of consciousness, above waking, dreaming and sleeping, stirs up fierce opposition as "unbounded" would mean the mind resides outside of the brain.

The way to prove the truth of unbounded consciousness is not by adding divine thought, not by persuading anyone who would believe that God is in the wings. It's more convincing to doctors especially if you direct them to the intimate scale of the human body. When somebody says, "Where's the mind?"They will point to their heads automatically. Why? For what? Is it because we simply allow our feelings to be heard in our heads? That's seemingly the case. This is a little more complex when dreaming at night, because we believe that we are "inside" our dreams. But for most of us, "my head" is mostly where "my mind" is located.

This response can just feel true because there are so many sensory organs: eyes, ears, nose, tongue. But the common sense model of sight and sound that takes place in the head can easily be undermined. When a car fires behind you, the sound cannot be felt as it enters the ear canal, is processed in the inner ear and then in the auditory center of the brain. There is no brain noise. The echo of the backfiring car comes very distinctly from outside of you. Hearing is a service in some cultures that moves from within to outside, the reverse of what we think. Dream of going down the highway and then seeing the driver hit the brakes in front of you. Your attention goes out to see the rear lights coming on. The senses are paying focus and makes it possible to suggest that when you saw the brake lights, your mind went beyond your body. If we suggest that someone "shoots a look" at someone else we implicitly follow this pattern for vision.

Babies, we are told, have a much more diffuse experience of the five senses, perhaps mixing them up into what are called synesthesias (for example, experiencing sounds as colors or tastes as shapes, an experience reported from hallucinogenic drugs, and in deep meditative states). Some researchers argue that thus, babies have a poor sense of the boundary between themselves and the world. Yet babies are children, and the distinction between themselves and the environment continues to harden. Society and family are reinforcing this pattern as the child grows up, and gradually the mind takes its seat in our minds, or so it seems. There are countless reports, repeated by Charles Lindbergh in his transatlantic flight, of altered states, whether caused by medication or in deep meditation, of the mind stretching in all directions. There are even anecdotal accounts of sitting in a chair and reaching out far across the room to touch those velvet drapes — the senses simply go where they are led.

Neuroscientists would call such experiences anomalies, resolutely declaring that mind and brain have taken up residence in a box called the skull together. But it is undeniably important to "think outside of the box" literally, beginning with the message system explored in this book that connects every cell in the body with whatever occurs in the brain. "Fine," would a neuroscientist argue, "but the brain is still the mind-making machine. Take the brain away, and there's no mind. "But this is the same as saying that there's no music when you turn off the radio. You didn't destroy the recording, just the receiver.

One must be open to questions that are historically revolutionary, including the most controversial of all: Is a brain really required for "thinking?" There are different ways of looking into this problem.

Next, let's consider how minds are formed by just human brains. Few people who have pets or work on farms will say there are no minds about the creatures they meet. There is already ample evidence that mammals have the DNA, neurons, and neurotransmitters involved in human brain function. It is not so disturbing to suggest that different kinds of animal brains build minds when you believe that the mind is embedded in these common mechanisms and chemicals. They can not explain what animal brains are like (some may lack something like human self-awareness), but we shouldn't have a difficulty conceiving that such animals have one.

Second, on the evolutionary ladder there are nervous systems that don't require a central brain. Some creatures have the neuronal nets distributed throughout the body, such as jellyfish. We have such systems as this too. The gastrointestinal tract sends and receives impulses from the peripheral nerves from the spinal cord that branch out. But when disconnected from the peripheral nervous system, digestion can function quite well. The intestine is a weblike digestive nervous system just like in the jellyfish. Specialized ganglion cells in the language of cell biology are located in the intestinal wall between muscle layers which act like a local brain. When one severs certain peripheral nerves, these ganglion cells tend to urge the intestine to pass, digest, and secrete, acting somewhat autonomously as a single entity embedded within itself.

The intestinal tract only takes advice from the rest of the body, it turns out. It harbors reactions of its own. When bad news in the pit of your stomach gives you a sinking feeling, you experience an emotion just as surely as you experience it in your head. In reality, the idea is followed by your gut reaction. Does that mean that your bowel nervous system creates these reactions on its own? That's unclear, but to think that way is tempting. Sure more people have faith in their gut reactions over the uncertain and unreliable responses that often burden the brain with.

The facial muscles are directly connected to your brain. While we assume the brain tells the mouth and lips to smile when we feel happy, the reverse is true, too. It can make you happy to see a smile on someone else's face, and children are taught to smile as a way to break out of a sad mood. Whether this happens or not varies from person to person but in those cases it could be argued that the face controls the brain.

Findings have become common on brain-like processes outside of the skull. The conductive structure inside the heart, like pacemaker cells, which organizes the heartbeat, can be known as the brain of the heart, just as the intestine's brain is the ganglion cells in the gut. Conduction system independence is shown when a transplanted heart continues to beat even though the nerves that connected it to the central and peripheral nervous systems of the donor have been severed. The interaction between the independent processing of the heart and that of the brain is complex and not fully understood.

The trillions of bacteria that outnumber the cells of the body by ten to one are even more enigmatic, residing mostly within the digestive tract but also on the skin and in the brain and other organs. We think of these bacteria as pests, but these micro-organisms were simply introduced in vast stretches along the double helix of human DNA over eons. The consequences are immense and essentially uncharted for what we call "being alive" The bacterial part of the body, taken as a whole, is called the microbiome. It is not sitting on the skin or in the gut passively, nor is it invading the body. Actually, the microbiota is the barrier between "in here" and "out there," containing DNA, antibodies, and chemical signaling that allows the brain to do the same stuff. There is no clear role of the microbial DNA that is incorporated into our genomes, but at least this is ancestral material that we have assimilated as our own. More suggestively, this once-foreign DNA in all higher life-forms may be the swapping mechanism for genes.

These discoveries demonstrate that our intelligence extends to the whole of ecology. Everywhere mentality has a physical basis. Any attempt at isolating it in the skull comes up against serious objections. Instead of treating cynicism with unbounded consciousness, we need to see that every perception is unbounded. By going beyond the illusory boundaries of the disconnected body, you cannot see, hear or touch anything in the universe. Watching a sunset is like watching yourself, actually.

The method causing phobias can be used to knock down a wall in exactly the opposite way, rather than build it. We should talk about people who resolve worries which are expected to be natural just as quickly, and far more happily. On skyscrapers, the construction workers used to include a large proportion of Mohawk Indians, who were raised without fear of heights. Practice can gradually build up the same courage into itself— for example, by walking a tightrope.

This versatility is not restricted to state psychology. Nutritionists have plenty of scientific evidence to show that the body needs to be given some vitamins and minerals on a daily basis to avoid falling victim to malnutrition diseases— the main instance being scurvy, which plagued the British navy while sailors were fed only on hardtack biscuits and deprived of vitamin C in fruits and vegetables.

Nevertheless, native cultures all over the world have lived without stringent daily vitamin standards for millennia and have adapted very well. In physiological circles the Tarahumara Indians of northern Sonora in Mexico have become famous because they can run twenty-five to fifty miles a day at high altitudes without discomfort. Whole tribes run these marathons every week; two minutes after crossing the finish line, when the winner of one race was checked, an American physiologist found that his heart rate was higher than when he stopped.

Which amplifies this extraordinary feat is that for the average family, half of which is made from corn milk, the Tarahumara typically live on two hundred pounds of corn a year. During the limited growing season other nutrition sources such as root vegetables become available in small quantities. Such people are showing the nearly infinite resilience of the mind-body system by being able to thrive on an absurdly understated diet. Ironically, their adaptation is so perfect that when placed on a "balanced" diet fortified with vitamins and minerals, many indigenous people develop epidemic proportions of heart disease, hypertension, skin disorders and rotten teeth, none of which they have had before.

Such definitions clearly pose a challenge to our whole understanding of what is natural. We have ample evidence within our own culture that our ability to create our own reality is what is most normal about us. It is incomprehensible that our thoughts can move molecules, as Sir John Eccles told the parapsychologists, and yet we live quite comfortably with this impossibility throughout. The rishis simply extend our comfort zone all the way, beyond limitless normality.

We already know that if an impulse of intelligence wants to do something, then it does it to find its outlet, using intellect, mind, senses and matter. Intelligence can create a physiology in which thoughts of healing take place but it can also create the reverse. If we were like a computer "hard-wired," then every physiology would be predictable; in reality, there is no physiology there. Intelligence creates new circuits at will which makes each individual unique. Any life experience changes the anatomy of the brain. The new dendrites that are created in active old people's brain cells are just one example.

The following experiment is even more extraordinary: Dr. Herbert Spector of the National Institutes of Health took a group of mice and gave them poly-I: C, a chemical believed to enhance the development of natural killer T-cells in the immune system, thus improving the protection of the animal against disease. Each time a mouse received its dose of poly-I: C, the camphor smell was released simultaneously in the vicinity.

The pattern continued for a few weeks, injecting the chemical and releasing the smell of a camphor. Spector exposed the mice only to the camphor when the chemical was taken away, and he found that their count of immune cells increased again, even without the chemical. In other words, they were made stronger by the smell alone against illness. Could he have done the reverse and a scent diminished their immunity?

Earlier a researcher at Rochester University proved this is true. They took a group of rats and fed them with cyclophosphamide, a chemical that is known to diminish immune response efficiency. At the same time, the rats were given saccharine-sweetened juice, which replaced the neutral agent for camphor. When the medication was removed, the animals also decreased their count of immune cells simply by degusting the water. What fascinated the researchers at the time was their understanding that the immune system has the ability to learn. It responds directly to stimuli from outside, not just to the bloodstream's internal environment.

Nevertheless, in a broader sense these studies warn us that the body is not bound to programmed reactions. A cell's Intelligence is innovative. The predictable mechanism that responds to poly-I: C positively and cyclophosphamide negatively can transform itself and respond to anything. It can also turn around and react with opposite results— the camphor scent could have been related to either drug.

There is no predetermined relation, though, between what type of experience you bring into the body and the outcome that comes out — your nervous system is set up for unboundedness. The more we focus on that, the more apparent are the consequences. The camphor scent did nothing to induce immune cell change: the mice might have eaten flowers or listened to a Mozart quartet. What actually happened between them was the development of an intuition instinct, a fully dynamic force co-ordinating a portion of the non-material world with a piece of the material world. This was very well known by the antique rishis. A verse from the Veda says, "You become what you see." In other words, the experience of perceiving the world just makes you what you are. This argument is quite direct. Children who grow up in homes where there is inadequate love may exhibit a variety of symptoms— they may be unhappy, neurotic, schizophrenic, sick, angry, or any number of other responses. But one of the most strange is a condition which is called psychosocial dwarfism. Such children do not grow up; they induce a deficiency of the pituitary growth hormone in themselves, and thus remain small and undeveloped in their physiques.

Ignoring the biological clock, it is possible to delay the onset of puberty; hence, the development of mental skills associated with older children, which is not directly controlled by the pituitary. It is not a pituitary disorder that is at fault, for when these kids are put in caring environments, their illness will change naturally, and they easily catch up with their peers in height.

Growing up is a built-in, genetically programmed birth outcome— yet these kids are defying it simply because they feel unloved. Even if the growth hormone is injected by a doctor many refuse to grow. A study conducted on adult male heart attack patients found that the most significant factor in their recovery — whether they survived or died — was nothing to do with food, exercise, alcohol, or a will to live. The men who lived thought their wives loved them while those who felt unloved appeared not to survive; no other connection was as significant as the researchers could discover.

The idea that every human may be an eternal being is now becoming more possible. Gifted with total versatility in our nervous systems, we all have the ability to create or tear down boundaries. That person constantly fabricates an endless number of emotions, experiences, wishes, things, etc. These impulses become your reality, rippling through the ocean of consciousness. If you knew how to control the creation of intelligence impulses, you could not just grow new dendrites but something else.

"What you see, you are" is a reality that forms the human body, even the brain. This was brought home by an innovative experiment developed by psychologists Joseph Hubel and David Weisel, with newborn kittens again involved. There were three sets of kittens put in carefully controlled conditions when they opened their eyes. The first was a white box painted with black horizontal stripes; the second was a white box painted with black vertical stripes; the third box was left empty.

After having been exposed to these conditions during the critical few days when sight evolved, the brains of the kittens conformed to them for life. The animals raised in a world with horizontal stripes could see nothing vertical correctly— they would run into chair legs, the verticality of which had little or no reality to them. The vertical-stripe box batch had exactly the opposite problem, being unable to see horizontal lines. The kittens from the all-white surroundings had a greater disorientation and could not respond correctly to any objects.

Such creatures were what they saw, because they now rigidly coded the neurons responsible for the sight. For humans too, the brain loses some of its unbounded intelligence whenever it perceives the universe across boundaries. That partial blindness remains inescapable without the ability to transcend. Impressions on our neurons are constantly being set for each of the senses, not just sight. Though we usually call the heavier impressions "stress," all impressions actually create some limitation.

For illustrate: In the early 1980s, M.I.T. experts began studying how human hearing function. Hearing seems passive, but in fact every person listens quite selectively to the world and puts his own interpretation on the raw data that comes into his ears. (For example, a skilled singer hears pitch and harmony where a tone-deaf person hears noise.) One experiment involves people listening to fast, basic rhythms (1-2-3 and 1-2-3 and 1-2-3), and teaching them to hear the rhythm differently (1, 2, 3-and-l, 2, 3-and-l, 2). After the noises started to be interpreted distinctly, the participants indicated that the sounds became more vibrant and fresher. The experiment evidently had taught people to change their unseen limits somewhat. The really interesting result, however, was that when they went home these people found the colours seemed lighter, music sounded better, the taste of food immediately became more pleasant, and everyone around them seemed lovable.

Just the slightest consciousness opening induced a change in reality. Meditation causes a bigger shift because it opens more channels of awareness and opens them to a deeper level. The shift does not separate us from the normal way we use our consciousness. Building borders will continue to be a fact of life. The twist provided by the rishis was to infuse this behavior with liberation, increasing it to a level which transcends the alienated ego's petty thoughts and desires. The ego typically has no choice but to actively waste life erecting one wall after another. It does this for the same reason as walls erected for the protection of medieval cities.

The ego considers the world a threatening, hostile place, for all that happens is different from the "I." This is the condition known as duality, and it's a great source of fear— the Veda calls it the only source of fear. Seeing "out there" we see all kinds of potential threats, all the stress and suffering that life can cause. The logical defense of the ego is to wall themselves in with the more friendly things— family, pleasures, happy memories, familiar places and activities. The rishis did not propose to tear down these territorial walls, though many people believe it was their intention to. The idea that Indian sages condemned the "illusion of life" took root in both East and West, and yet, Vedic reality was not based on such an absurdity.

Duality does exist, and recognition of a higher unity is made meaningful because of its existence. Two polar opposites combine into a whole — this idea gives a proper perspective on the quiet and active aspects of creation. When the rishis find peace, the silent field of knowledge, they found another pole which completes life. The ancient texts describe this as Purnam adah, purnam idam—"This is complete, that's full. "Then the highest goal of creation is to attain" two hundred per cent of life. "This can be achieved by the human nervous system because it is fluid enough to understand both the diversity of life, which is limitless yet free of limits, and the single world, which is similarly infinite but completely unbound. There could be no other possibility just from a logical standpoint. No one was given a celestial machine and said, "Mind, you can only use half of it." No one gave us any restrictions on the knowledge patterns that we can create, alter, combine, extend, and occupy. Living is a world with limitless possibilities. Such is the glory of absolute nervous system versatility in humans.

That is an enormously important issue. This says we should skip the tight, bounded choices we're used to making and go straight to solving any problem. The justification for this claim is that the solution of our consciousness is already formed by definition. The challenges are in the integration field whilst the solutions are in the unity field. Going straight to the area of harmony immediately reaches the solution which is then worked out by the mind-body system — that was the shortcut for the rishis.

Research on mortality by Robert Keith Wallace are an excellent example of how the shortcut works. The current scientific wisdom argues that aging is a complicated area which is poorly understood. Gerontology, the science of old age, became a discipline only since the 1950s, when the decoding of DNA made it possible to believe that there could be specific genes for aging (none have existed so far, although it is understood that certain aging pathways are genetically coded in lower animals). Now that gerontology is in high gear, it's swamped by conflicting theories and huge data banks collected from research projects which will take decades to complete.

This intensive research effort didn't make aging more slowly. The major advance in the field has been documenting that healthy people do not have to automatically deteriorate as they grow older, a point that has been made without databases for centuries. Gerontology has had some important medical applications, such as the recognition that many senile signs are reversible once assumed to be lifelong. They are not signs of brain decline but are the by-product of poor nutrition, isolation, dehydration and other factors in the environment of the individual. Alternatively, gerontology advances bit by bit, forming tiny connections in hypotheses that are, to begin with, conjectural. As for encouraging the American people to eat better, exercise sensibly, and pursue disease prevention, the entire field shares with the rest of the drugs.

However, Wallace's research proceeded on the assumption that people are aging not by bits and pieces but as human beings as a whole. Consequently, ageing contains a large option dimension. When old people will maintain their mental faculties by using them constantly, then the practice of meditation, which fully unlocks the mind, can do even more. As mentioned earlier, Wallace's basic observation was that long-term meditators had their biological age lowered by five to twelve years. (High levels of an unknown hormone called DHEA[dehydroepiandrosterone] have also been found; it has been hypothesized that DHEA somehow helps slow aging and may prevent cancer development and growth.) This research suggests that aging is regulated by consciousness. Operating at the usual level of shallow, confused thinking, we intensify the aging process of our bodies, but as we step into the transcendent area of quiet movement, mental activity ceases, and cell activity evidently responds accordingly. If this is true, then ageing can be programmed from different awareness levels. When we program to deteriorate ourselves, which was the norm in previous generations, then that becomes the truth. This kind of programming is not simply a matter of reasoning or believing. Positive attitudes, mental alertness, willingness to survive and other psychological characteristics can ease old age; they certainly help to crack the rigid social conditioning that often traps old people. Yet reversing the aging process itself is simply another, much deeper issue.

Officially, gerontology does not recognize any means of reversing or retarding the aging process— a rather strict position, if you consider that aging has not even been properly defined. The rishis would counter that science has failed to reach the awareness level where aging can be defeated. A young Harvard psychologist, Charles Alexander, went into three old-age homes outside Boston in 1980 and taught some mind-body techniques to about sixty residents, all at least 80 years old. Three were used: a mainstream relaxation technique (the kind used in typical stress management programs), Transcendental Meditation, and a set of creative word games to keep the mind sharp every day.

Each person learned only one technique and was permitted to use it without oversight by the classes. The meditators scored the highest on tests of increased cognitive capacity, low blood pressure, and mental health, all of which should decrease with age, when the three classes were assessed on follow-up. The people have also reported feeling better and not as tired as before. But not until three years later did the profoundly surprising outcome come to light. About one-third of the tenants had died after he left before Alexander returned to the old-age homes, including 24 percent of the people who had not practiced meditation. Nevertheless, the death rate was zero amongst the meditative community.

Those individuals had now lived at an average age of 84, one of the rarest and most amazing times when science conducted an experiment that bestowed the gift of life automatically. While limited in scope, this is one of the most promising results in the entire aging sector and a win for the path to the rishis. It says it's enough to increase your consciousness to prolong your career. What is the life span of meditators who started in their twenties rather than their eighties? Time will tell.

CONCLUSION

Now that you understand what Quantum healing is, you should continue using it every day.

Start by making sure that it is available first. Follow the simple steps in this book and see your life changing for the better. With you being more aware of those around you, you will feel confident in pursuing these tasks and connecting with different individuals. This is mostly because of the innate skill Quantum healing can warn you when certain acts are likely to harm you, and when others are likely to succeed.

You can increase your spiritual awareness and put into practice your learned abilities so that you can make a positive impact in your life and the people around you. Quantum healing is beneficial because it gives you the emotional awareness so you can live your normal life without getting overwhelmed.

Use this book as a reference and incorporate it into your daily routine and it sure to improve your life. Read this book everywhere, every time and let every word in this book be a part of you as you wake up in the morning, go to the gym, go to work and have a peaceful nigh rest. The words imbedded here are sure to make you feel excited and optimistic as you do about with your daily activities.

Get to the innate level that you were meant to be and don't hesitate to be congratulate yourself when you finally get your intuitive knowledge.